Diabetes Therapies
treating hyperglycaemia

Clifford J. Bailey
PhD, FRCP(Edin), FRCPath
Professor of Clinical Science
Aston University
Birmingham, UK

Michael D. Feher
MB BS, MD, FRCP
Consultant Physician in Diabetes
and Clinical Pharmacology
Chelsea and Westminster Hospital
London, UK

MedEd UK Ltd

i

Diabetes Therapies
treating hyperglycaemia

Clifford J Bailey and Michael D Feher

Published by MedEd UK Ltd,
Coombs Wood Centre, PO Box 11892, Halesowen, B63 8WE, UK.

© MedEd UK Ltd, 2009

ISBN 978-0-9563857-0-3

Layout and design: Heron Press
Photographic images: Andrew V Bailey and David J Bailey
Figures: Clifford J Bailey

Printed in Times New Roman by
Heron Press, Rubery, Birmingham B45 9AL, UK.

PREFACE

Diabetes Therapies is a guide to the use of blood glucose-lowering agents in the treatment of diabetes mellitus in the UK. As the epidemic of diabetes continues to escalate, more healthcare professionals, specialists and non-specialists, have become involved in the management of diabetes. Good glycaemic control is increasingly acknowledged as an essential pillar of long-term diabetes care, and several new drugs have recently joined the established medicines to address hyperglycaemia.

Here we try to provide a concise and practical reference that covers key information about these agents: how they work, their suitability and exclusions for different groups of patients, choosing and titrating the dose, monitoring and minimising the risk of interactions and adverse events.

People with diabetes, particularly type 2 diabetes, often require multiple therapies, frequent dose adjustments and alterations to their drug regimen to address disease progression. This is additional to prophylactic medication for cardiovascular risk and co-morbid conditions. Thus the management process is complex, varied and fraught with medicinal conundrums. This book assumes a general knowledge of diabetes and its management, and we hope it will provide ready access to content in a convenient format.

Clifford J Bailey
Michael D Feher

July 2009

CONTENTS

ABBREVIATIONS

ACE	angiotensin converting enzyme
ACS	acute coronary syndrome
ALT	alanine transaminase
aP2	adipocyte fatty acid binding protein-2
ARB	angiotensin receptor blocker
ATP	adenosine triphosphate
bd	*bis die*, twice daily
BMI	body mass index
BNF	British National Formulary
BP	blood pressure
Ca	calcium
CHO	carbohydrate
CrCl	creatinine clearance
CRP	C-reactive protein
CV	cardiovascular
CVD	cardiovascular disease
DAFNE	Dose Adjustment For Normal Eating
DBP	diastolic blood pressure
DESMOND	Diabetes Education and Self-Management for Ongoing and Newly Diagnosed
DKA	diabetic ketoacidosis
DPP4i	dipeptidyl peptidase-4 inhibitor
eGFR	estimated glomerular filtration rate
ESRD	end stage renal disease
FATP	fatty acid transporter protein (CD36)
FDC	fixed-dose combination
FFA	free fatty acid
FPG	fasting plasma glucose
G-6-Pase	glucose-6-phosphatase
GAD65	glutamic acid decarboxylase 65
GDA	guideline daily allowance
GDM	gestational diabetes mellitus
GI	gastrointestinal
GIP	gastric inhibitory polypeptide
GLP-1	glucagon-like peptide-1
GLUT	glucose transporter,
GP	general practitioner
HbA1c	glycated haemoglobin
HDLc	high-density lipoprotein cholesterol
HGO	hepatic glucose output
HLA	human leucocyte antigen
HONK	hyperosmolar non-ketotic
HSD-1	hydroxysteroid dehydrogenase-1
Hypo	episode of hypoglycaemia
IDDM	insulin-dependent diabetes mellitus
IFG	impaired fasting glucose
IGF-1	insulin-like growth factor-1
IGT	impaired glucose tolerance
IL-6	interleukin-6
IMT	intima-media thickness
INR	international normalised ratio
iv	intravenous
JOD	juvenile-onset diabetes
K	potassium
K$^+$ATP	ATP-sensitive potassium channel Kir6.2

Abbreviations

Kir6.2	potassium inward rectifying channel 6.2
kcal	kilocalorie
kJ	kilojoule
LADA	latent autoimmune diabetes in adults
LDLc	low-density lipoprotein cholesterol
LPL	lipoprotein lipase
MCP-1	monocyte chemoattractant protein-1
MDI	multiple daily injections (of insulin)
MDRD	Modification of Diet in Renal Disease
mg	milligram (10^{-3} g)
MI	myocardial infarction
MMP-9	matrix metalloproteinase-9
MOD	maturity onset diabetes
MODY	maturity onset diabetes of the young
NAFLD	non-alcoholic fatty liver disease
NASH	non-alcoholic steatohepatitis
NFKB	nuclear factor kappa-B
NICE	National Institute for Health and Clinical Excellence
NIDDM	non-insulin-dependent diabetes mellitus
NSAID	non-steroidal anti-inflammatory drug
NYHA	New York Heart Association
OAT3	organic anion transporter-3
OAD	oral antidiabetic agent
Oct1	organic cation transporter-1
od	*omni die*, once daily, every day
OGTT	oral glucose tolerance test
OTC	over the counter
P	pharmacy supplied
PAI-1	plasminogen activator inhibitor-1
PCOS	polycystic ovary syndrome
POM	prescription only medicine
PPAR	peroxisome proliferator-activated receptor
PPG	postprandial plasma glucose
QOF	Quality and Outcomes Framework
RBP	retinol binding protein
RXR	retinoid-X-receptor
SBP	systolic blood pressure
sc	subcutaneous
SMBG	self-monitoring of blood glucose
SNRI	serotonin and noradrenaline re-uptake inhibitor
SPC	summary of product characteristics
SUR1	sulphonylurea receptor-1
SUR2A/B	sulphonylurea receptor-2A/B
T1DM	type 1 diabetes mellitus
T2DM	type 2 diabetes mellitus
tds	*ter die sumendum*, to be taken three times daily
TC	total cholesterol
TG	triglycerides
TIA	transient ischaemic attack
TNFα	tumour necrosis factor-alpha
TZD	thiazolidinedione
UCP1	uncoupling protein-1
μg	microgram (10^{-6} g)
UKPDS	United Kingdom Prospective Diabetes Study
ULN	upper limit of normal
WHR	waist-to-hip ratio
↓ Decrease	
↑ Increase	

1 DIABETES INTRODUCTION

Definition

Diabetes mellitus describes a group of metabolic diseases characterised by hyperglycaemia, resulting from defects in insulin secretion, insulin action, or both. The chronic hyperglycaemia of diabetes is associated with long-term damage, dysfunction and failure of various organs, especially the eyes, kidneys, nerves, heart, and blood vessels (Expert Committee on Diagnosis and Classification, 1997).

Table 1.1 Types of diabetes

Type 1 diabetes

Insulin-dependent diabetes mellitus, IDDM
Ketosis–prone diabetes
(formerly juvenile-onset diabetes)

Type 2 diabetes

Non-insulin-dependent diabetes mellitus, NIDDM
(formerly maturity-onset diabetes)

Gestational diabetes

Diabetes emerging in pregnancy, GDM

MODY

Maturity Onset Diabetes of the Young
(sometimes called monogenic diabetes)

Other forms of diabetes

Drug-induced
    eg. glucocorticoids, thiazides, beta-blockers
Genetic defects of insulin action
    eg. Leprechaunism
Pancreatic conditions
    Pancreatitis and other exocrine pancreatic diseases
Endocrinopathies
    eg. Cushing's disease, acromegaly
Rare genetic syndromes
    eg. Down's, Prader-Willi

Prevalence

Diabetes mellitus affects >4% of people in the UK (>2.3 million). In 2005-6, the prevalence of diabetes amongst people registered with GP practices was 3.6% in England, and 4.1% in Wales. Screening studies have shown that about 1% of the population has diabetes that is undiagnosed. The occurrence of type 1 and type 2 diabetes is increasing, and the prevalence is projected to exceed 5% of the UK population by 2020.

Type 1 diabetes has a prevalence in children, <18 yrs, in England of about 200 per 100,000. The incidence is increasing, especially amongst the under fives. New cases in children <18 yrs appear to be increasing by 2-3% per year.

Type 2 diabetes, which accounts for 90-95% of all cases of diabetes, is more common with advancing adult age (>6% of people over 60 years): this appears to be associated with the increased occurrence of obesity. Most ethnic minority groups in the UK are at increased risk of type 2 diabetes, and there is an emerging occurrence of type 2 diabetes in children.

Type 1 diabetes

The cause of type 1 diabetes appears (but is not actually proven) to result from prior exposure to viruses in genetically susceptible individuals. This initiates an autoimmune destruction of β-cells which may occur over months or years (decades in a few individuals). When >90% of β-cells are destroyed the remaining β-cells are unable to maintain glucose homeostasis, and patients often present with marked hyperglycaemia eg. blood glucose >25 mmol/L (450 mg/dL).

Without insulin, the body is unable to utilise glucose, so fat is mobilised as an energy source. Excess fat metabolism generates ketones, hence ketoacidosis. Protein may also be used as an energy source, causing emaciation in severely affected and untreated patients. When treatment is implemented there is a 'honeymoon period' of improved wellbeing, but within a matter of months most if not all β-cells are lost, necessitating absolute reliance on insulin therapy.

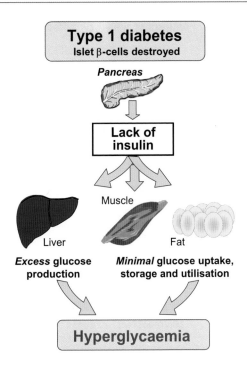

Figure 1.1   Type 1 diabetes mellitus – route to hyperglycaemia
Destruction of β-cells in the islets of Langerhans in the pancreas
causes an absolute lack of insulin.   Without insulin there is a
marked excess production of glucose by the liver and much
diminished uptake of glucose by muscle.   This results in very
severe hyperglycaemia.   An absolute lack of insulin is acutely
fatal.

Type 2 diabetes

Most patients incur a gradual loss of insulin sensitivity (ie onset
of insulin resistance) over a decade or more of adult life before
development of diabetes. Obesity and increased lipid
accumulation in muscle and liver cells exacerbate this process.
During this time insulin secretion usually increases to
compensate, but detrimental changes in β-cell function such as

Table 1.2 Features of type 1 diabetes mellitus

Acronyms	T1DM, IDDM (formerly JOD)
Age of onset	Mostly <20yrs May occur later (eg. LADA, latent autoimmune diabetes in adults)
Occurrence	~5 – 10 % of all diabetes Incidence per 100,000 children per year is 10-20 in England and >20 in Scotland
Hyperglycaemia	Severe and fatal if untreated
Ketosis and coma	Ketoacidosis and coma if untreated
Pancreatic β-cells	All destroyed: usually T-cell mediated autoimmune process; occasionally toxic chemicals or idiopathic
Insulin secretion	Absolute loss of insulin: most patients produce no endogenous insulin (C-peptide negative)
Insulin resistance	No (but may develop with insulin therapy)
Complications	Microvascular: common Macrovascular: modest increase in risk
Treatment	Insulin replacement therapy essential Lifestyle - diet and exercise adjustments required
Genetics	Family history of diabetes in <10% of cases Probably polygenic susceptibility, variable penetrance
HLA association	Strong association: DQA, DQB and DRB
Antibodies	Autoantibodies to islet cells, insulin and GAD65 in >80% of patients at diagnosis
Environmental	Probably triggered by viruses (eg. mumps, coxsackie) and chemical toxins
Hypoglycaemia	Very susceptible – review insulin therapy. Treat with glucose or glucagon

Table 1.3 Features of type 2 diabetes mellitus

Acronyms	T2DM, NIDDM (formerly MOD)
Age of onset	Mostly >40yrs May occur earlier, especially in obese individuals.
Occurrence	~90 – 95 % of all diabetes Present in >6% of people >60 yrs old. Much higher prevalence in South Asians
Hyperglycaemia	Usually moderate and not acutely fatal
Ketosis and coma	Non-ketotic coma (HONK); ketosis rare
Pancreatic β-cells	Dysfunctional: insulin responses initially delayed but extended, diminishing as disease progresses. Reduced β-cell mass.
Insulin secretion	Relative insulin deficiency: some endogenous insulin secretion remaining, decreasing with disease progression
Insulin resistance	Yes, may be severe in some patients
Complications	Microvascular: common Macrovascular: marked increase in risk
Treatment	Lifestyle (diet, exercise) recommended Oral and injectable agents and/or insulin usually required
Genetics	Family history of diabetes in 40-80% of cases. Polygenic: affecting insulin action, energy metabolism, and β-cell function
HLA association	No apparent association with HLA genes
Antibodies	Rarely any evidence of antibodies to islet cells or insulin
Environmental	Obesity (BMI >30 kg/m^2) for 10 yrs increases risk >10 fold vs BMI <22 kg/m^2
Hypoglycaemia	Susceptible if treated with insulin or some insulin secretagogues. Treat with glucose

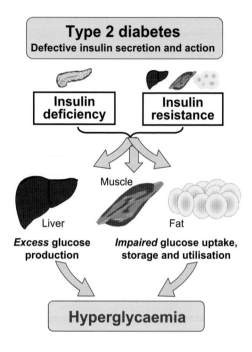

Figure 1.2 Type 2 diabetes mellitus – route to hyperglycaemia
Insulin resistance (impaired cellular action of insulin) and islet
β-cell dysfunction (delayed and/or reduced insulin secretion)
cause a relative lack of insulin. The combination of insulin
resistance and β-cell dysfunction allows excess glucose
production by the liver and diminished glucose metabolism by
muscle. This results in moderate hyperglycaemia. The insulin
resistance, modest hyperglycaemia and associated metabolic and
vascular disturbances contribute to chronic morbidity and
premature mortality.

loss of the first phase insulin response to glucose result in delayed
insulin secretion after a meal.

Other defects of β-cell function such as an increased
proportion of proinsulin (which is less effective than insulin)
contribute to an impairment of glucose homeostasis.

When the β-cells can no longer meet the increased demand for insulin, hyperglycaemia emerges and increases progressively, and overt diabetes develops as β-cell function continues to decline. Over-production of glucagon by pancreatic α-cells adds to the hyperglycaemia through increased hepatic glucose production.

MODY and other forms of diabetes

MODY is due to genetic defects of pancreatic β-cell function, mostly caused by autosomal dominant mutations of genes encoding glucokinase, certain hepatic nuclear factors or other transcription factors.

Diabetes can also develop in some rare genetic conditions, or associated with pancreatic diseases or various drugs.

Presenting features of diabetes

At diagnosis there is usually a history of fatigue, thirst, polyuria, visual disturbances and quite often recent weight loss.

Type 1 diabetes

Type 1 patients are not commonly obese, although obesity may hasten onset and complicate diagnosis and treatment. Patients seldom present with the emaciation seen in the past. A history of non-specific failure to thrive is often noted in younger children, despite good appetite and no evidence of neglect. A recent illness that is likely to escalate symptoms may be described. Occasional presentation occurs in ketoacidosis, usually with nausea or vomiting, dehydration, abdominal discomfort, hyperventilation and impaired consciousness.

Type 2 diabetes

Type 2 patients are commonly overweight or obese, or recount a history of such. Many are brought to attention by a cardiovascular event, persistent infection, random screening or insurance medicals. At least one quarter of patients will exhibit complications at the time of diagnosis indicating that the condition has existed undiagnosed for several years.

Predisposing factors

The genetic and environmental factors that confer susceptibility to and trigger the onset of type 1 diabetes are still unestablished. However, several risk factors have been identified for type 2 diabetes.

Table 1.4 Risk factors for type 2 diabetes mellitus

Parent or sibling with type 2 diabetes

Ethnicity, especially South Asian or Hispanic

Obesity (especially visceral) or history of prolonged overweight

Advancing adult age

IGT or IFG

Other features of 'metabolic syndrome' (dyslipidaemia, raised BP)

Certain other endocrinopathies (eg acromegaly, Cushing's disease)

Receiving diabetogenic drug therapy (eg, glucocorticoids, thiazides, beta-blockers)

Sedentary lifestyle

Gestational diabetes that resolved after pregnancy

Very low or very high birth weight

Cigarette smoking

Complications

The microvascular (retinopathy, nephropathy) and neuropathic complications of diabetes can mostly be attributed to the 'glucotoxicity' of prolonged hyperglycaemia. The macrovascular complications strongly reflect co-existent dyslipidaemia, insulin resistance, hypertension and hypercoagulation which affect the predisposition to athero-thrombotic disease.

Table 1.5 Complications of diabetes mellitus

Mortality

Life expectancy	Decreased 5–10 years[a]
Fatal coronary heart disease	Increased 2– 4 fold
Fatal stroke	Increased 2–3 fold

Morbidity

Coronary heart disease	Increased 2–3 fold
Cerebrovascular disease	Increased > 2 fold
Peripheral vascular disease	Increased 2–3 fold
Retinopathy (over lifetime)	Affects about 80% of patients
Retinopathy (registered blind)	~1% of patients
Nephropathy (proteinuria)	Affects 5–30% of patients
Neuropathy (over lifetime)	Affects about 60% of patients
Hypertension (over lifetime)	Affects >60% of patients
Lower limb amputation	Increased several fold
Depression	Increased 2 fold

[a] depending on age at diagnosis. The macrovascular complications are noted for type 2 diabetes: they are generally less in type 1 diabetes.

Costs

The detrimental effect of diabetes on quality of life is immense. It also impacts the lives of family, friends and work colleagues, for example employment may be lost, lifestyle radically altered and personal costs for healthcare increased. Diabetes increases hospitalisation, GP visits and drug use, and accounts for approaching 10% of direct healthcare costs in the UK.

The indirect and intangible costs of diabetes are beyond accurate quantification.

Diagnosis of diabetes

The diagnosis of diabetes and the categories of sub-diabetic hyperglycaemia are based on venous plasma (or blood) glucose taken at random, or in the fasted state, or at 2h after a 75g oral glucose tolerance test (OGTT). Glucose measurements should be repeated if the person is asymptomatic, and one measurement should be made by a recognised laboratory.

Table 1.6 Diagnostic criteria for diabetes mellitus, IGT and IFG

	Plasma glucose	
	mmol/L	mg/dL
Diabetes		
Random	≥11.1	≥200
Fasting	≥7.0	≥126
2h 75g OGTT	≥11.1	≥200
IGT		
2h 75g OGTT	7.8-11.0	140-199
IFG		
Fasting	>6.0-<7.0	>110-<126

Metabolic syndrome

When considering the care of the newly diagnosed type 2 diabetic patient it is important to assess cardiovascular risk, and to identify any existing or emerging risk factors.

Type 2 diabetes is commonly associated with a cluster of cardiovascular risk factors. These are known as the 'metabolic syndrome' and several of the factors are usually found in the same individual, and presence of one or more should prompt checks for others. The exact defining features of the syndrome are not agreed but the main components are recognised in several attempted definitions.

Table 1.7 Metabolic syndrome

Component	WHO	NCEP (ATP III)	IDF
Insulin resistance	Present	Not essential	Not essential
Hyperglycaemia IFG, 2h IGT (mmol/L) or T2DM	IFG ≥6.1 or IGT ≥7.8 or T2DM	IFG ≥6.1	IFG ≥ 5.6 or Rx
Central obesity Waist (cm) or WHR or BMI (kg/m²)	WHR >0.9 (>0.85) BMI >30	Waist >102 (>88)	Waist >94 (>80)*
Raised BP (mmHg)	≥140/90	≥130/85	≥130/85 or Rx
Raised TG (mmol/L)	≥1.7	≥1.7	≥1.7 or Rx
Low HDLc (mmol/L)	<0.9 (1.0)	<1.04 (<1.29)	<1.03 (≥1.29) or Rx
Number of components for diagnosis	IR or IFG or IGT plus ≥2 others from: central obesity (using WHR and /or BMI), raised BP, dyslipidaemia (raised TG +/- raised HDLc) or microalbumuria	≥3 of the components above	Central obesity (waist circumference) plus 2 other components. Waist circumference defined for different ethnic groups

Metabolic syndrome describes a clustering of cardiovascular risk factors, several or all of which often occur in the same individual. Type 2 diabetes, IGT and IFG are components of the syndrome. Different expert groups have proposed slightly different diagnostic criteria

WHO, World Health Organisation; NCEP (ATP III), National Cholesterol Education Program (Adult Treatment Panel III), IDF, International Diabetes Federation; IR, insulin resistance; Rx, receiving treatment;
* waist measurements for Europids; ( ), values for women in parentheses

Table 1.8 Components of a diabetes care plan

Immediate action:
>Refer if required, especially for type 1 diabetes
>Manage existing symptoms and complications
>Undertake further investigations as appropriate

Additional Action:
>Provide advice on living with diabetes
>Start education for patient empowerment
>Start lifestyle intervention
>Start antidiabetic drug therapy if required
>Assess other medication needs (eg. for CV risk)
>Organise contact with other members of care team
>Establish review schedule

Care plan

After diagnosis, a thorough clinical and general review should provide the basis for an individualised care plan. This will address the particular needs and circumstances of the patient.

For type 1 diabetes the plan will involve immediate referral to a specialist to start insulin. Care plans will be shaped by local protocols and facilities, service agreements and commissioning.

However every care plan should initiate action to relieve symptoms, start the long-term treatment programme and engage the patient in education and empowerment to contribute effectively in their own disease management.

2 LIFESTYLE MANAGEMENT

Lifestyle factors

Lifestyle is fundamental to every diabetes management programme. It includes an appreciation of:
* Diet
* Exercise
* Body weight control
* Healthy living advice
* 'Living with diabetes'

Diet

People with diabetes should follow a normal healthy diet. The amount of food and timing of meals and snacks should be consistent with daily routine, antidiabetic drug therapy and other medications, as well as extra physical activity and desired body weight control. People are generally encouraged to:

Reduce   - saturated fat, simple sugars, salt, alcohol,

Maintain - complex CHO, fibre, vitamins, minerals and water unless there are good reasons to do otherwise (eg. the water-diuretic debate).

Carbohydrate

Complex carbohydrate such as bread, cereals, potatoes, rice and pasta, along with legumes and pulses will normally form the major energy component and a major source of fibre. The slow rate of digestion reduces the rate at which glucose enters the circulation and lowers the extent of the glycaemic excursion.

Fat

Due to links with cardiovascular disease, diets should be low in saturated (animal) fats and *trans*-fatty acids (eg. deep-fried foods and margarine). Other types of fats, including mono- and polyunsaturated vegetable oils and n-3 fatty acids in fish oils are recommended in moderation.

Table 2.1 Proposed healthy diet composition

Component	Amount	Suggest
Carbohydrate	>55% total energy	<25g/day added sugar <50g/day total sugar
Fat	<30% total energy	<10% saturated 10-15% mono-unsaturated <10% polyunsaturated
Protein	10-15% total energy	
Fibre	>30g/day	
Salt	<6g/day	<3g/day if hypertensive
Cholesterol	<300mg/day	
Vitamins	≥ GDA	Within normal foods
Minerals	≥ GDA	Within normal foods
Alcohol	<30g/day	≤ 2 glasses of red wine

Protein

Meat, fish and pulses are the main sources of protein, but bread, some dairy products (eg. low-fat cheese) and many vegetables are a valuable source of protein. Some authorities suggest a suitable daily amount of protein is about 0.8 g/kg body weight.

Vitamins and minerals

While the 'five-a-day' portions of fruit and vegetables should supply adequate vitamins and minerals, people with diabetes often have sub-normal circulating concentrations of some vitamins and minerals, commonly magnesium, chromium, iron, and vitamin D. There is some evidence that replacement (but not supra-normal supplementation) amounts of these substances (eg. with a low-dose multivitamin-mineral supplement) can be beneficial.

Cholesterol and salt

In the interests of macrovascular protection, the amount of dietary cholesterol (eg. egg yolk) and salt should be limited.

Fibre

A normal diet should contain adequate fibre, but fibre-rich foods such as cereals and pulses may need to be encouraged. To help slow the digestion and absorption of nutrients, fibre supplements may have a small effect. These include soluble fibre such as guar gum (E412; a galactomannan from the Indian cluster bean) or fruit pectins, and insoluble fibre such as wheat bran and cellulose.

Alcohol

Alcohol is a rich source of calories. It also interferes with the hepatic metabolism of some antidiabetic drugs and other medications taken by diabetic patients. Very importantly, alcohol can inhibit hepatic gluconeogenesis. This increases the risk and enhances the severity of hypoglycaemia occurring with antidiabetic drugs.

Energy content

A typical modest daily diet will comprise about 2000 kcal (8400 kJ) of energy. The basal metabolic rate (ie. metabolism at rest) might be expected to use about 1500 kcal (6300 kJ), allowing 500 kcal (2100 kJ) for voluntary physical activity. Thus someone who is inactive would typically require a daily intake of less than 2000 kcal (8400 kJ) to lose weight.

Reducing daily intake by about 500 kcal (2100 kJ) will usually achieve weight loss. Note that fat is 2¼ times more energy dense than carbohydrate or protein: thus a reduction in fat intake can be conveniently helpful for weight reduction and dietary composition in overweight patients. Fad diets and speciality foods do not appear to offer extra benefits.

Table 2.2 Energy content of foods and examples of amounts consumed in a recommended 1500 kcal or 2000 kcal diet

	Energy	1500 kcal diet			2000 kcal diet		
	kcal/g[a] (kJ/g)	g[b]	kcal[a]	%[c]	g[b]	kcal[a]	%[c]
Carbohydrate	4 (17)	225	900	60	295	1180	59
Fat	9 (38)	40	360	24	60	540	27
Protein	4 (17)	60	240	16	70	280	14

[a] 1 kcal = 4.2 kJ; values in parenthesis are kJ/g
[b] g = gram; oz = ounce; 1g = 0.035oz; 1oz = 28.3g
[c] % energy content of diet

Exercise

The cardiovascular and metabolic benefits of aerobic exercise are well recognised, as well as their value for reducing adiposity and building muscle tone.

Table 2.3 Energy expenditure during exercise*

Exercise	Duration per bout (minutes)	Bouts per day	Energy expended kcal/hr
Normal walking (2.5 miles/h)	30	1-2	140-200
Brisk walking (3-4 miles/h)	15-30	1-2	200-300
Jogging (5miles/h)	10-20	1	~500
Leisure cycling	10-20	1	300-500
Leisure swimming	10-20	1	300-500
Gardening	15-60	1-2	100-250
Housework	15-60	1-3	~100

*Typical realistic target levels of exercise recommended for a previously sedentary adult without contraindications, showing approximate amounts of energy expended for a non-obese person

Exercise programmes should be structured to:
- Build up gradually
- Set realistic targets
- Harmonise with drug and diet therapy
- Avoid hypoglycaemia
- Avoid foot damage

Contraindications must be recognised and respected, especially cardiovascular, pulmonary and osteo-arthritic disorders.

Body weight and adiposity

Body mass index (BMI) is the standard surrogate measure for overweight and obesity, and waist circumference is sometimes used as a rough indication of intra-abdominal adiposity. Waist-to-hip ratio (WHR) is also used as a surrogate for abdominal obesity.

$$\text{Body mass index} \quad = \quad \frac{\text{weight} \quad (\text{kg})}{\text{height} \quad (\text{m}^2)}$$

Table 2.4 Clinical measures of body weight and obesity for Europids*

	BMI (kg/m^2)
Underweight	<18.5
Normal	18.5-24.9
overweight	25-29.9
Obese	≥30
Extreme obesity	≥40

*For people from South Asia consider BMI overweight >23 and obese >28 for similar cardiovascular risk

Intra-abdominal fat

Intra-abdominal (visceral) adiposity is particularly detrimental as it is strongly associated with increased risk of CV disease, and strongly predicts the development of diabetes, even when overall body weight is not excessive. Visceral fat produces certain adipokines and has a high turnover of lipids that could account for this.

Table 2.5 Normal values of waist circumference and waist-to-hip ratio for Europids

	Men	Women
Waist circumference	<94 cm (37 inches)	<88 cm (34.5 inches)
Waist-to-hip ratio	<0.95	<0.8

Body weight control

The act of attempting to lose weight (by dieting and exercise), and actually losing weight are all associated with improved metabolic control and improved outcomes. Reductions in 5-10% of body weight are considered realistic and clinically significant for an overweight individual, and >10% if possible for an obese person.

Weight loss is notoriously more difficult to achieve and sustain for people with diabetes due to the improved insulin sensitivity and a consequent increase in the anabolic effects of insulin. When patients are exercising a levelling out of body weight may still be beneficial as a continuing reduction in adipose mass may be disguised by increased muscle mass.

Weight reducing strategies

Combination of reduced energy intake (dieting) and increased output (exercise) is often more successful and safer than extremes of each individually.

A minimal (but realistic) approach is to reduce energy intake by about 500 kcal/day (eg. from 2500 to 2000 kcal/day) and to increase exercise by 1 moderate bout/day (eg. normal walking for 30 min expends 70-100 kcal). This approach might be expected to reduce body weight by about 0.5 kg/month for 6 months, and continue to reduce weight by 0.5 kg every 2 months to 24 months.

Note that metabolic efficiency increases with continued dieting, which reduces the rate of weight loss.

Healthy living advice

To facilitate change, provide advice on diet, exercise and weight control within the context of the patient's current lifestyle.

Table 2.6 Strategies to encourage a diet reduced by 500 kcal/day

Reduce all portions by one fifth

Quit or reduce alcohol

Stop unnecessary snacks

Use artificial sweeteners/low-calorie drinks

Choose more bulky foods

Trim surface fat from meat

Grill, don't fry

Encourage social activities – including membership of support groups - and strategies to minimise stress.

Inform on access to other healthcare professionals. Empathy with patient's perceived barriers may be used to initiate self-determination and empowerment to implement and maintain healthy lifestyle strategies.

Living with diabetes

Helping newly diagnosed patients coming to terms with a life-long condition may require very different and individualised forms of support. Being aware of personal circumstances and exploring opportunities to engage families and close social contacts can profoundly influence the manner in which patients view and manage their diabetes. It is important for everyone to appreciate that a healthy lifestyle and attention to 'good control' will reduce the risk of complications and minimise impact on daily life.

Access to a health psychologist and dietician, and participation in a dedicated programme such as DAFNE/DESMOND can be highly beneficial. Bringing a friend, providing reading material, visiting useful websites, contacting support groups, meeting other (expert) patients and having access to healthcare professionals are all valuable approaches to 'enabling' effective self-participation in the management process.

Weight (kg) → (top row values) / **Weight (lbs)** → (bottom row values)

Height (feet and inches) / **Height (metres)**

Height (feet and inches)	Height (metres)	114	109	105	100	95	91	86	82	77	73	68	64	59	55	50
6'2"	1.8	32	31	30	28	27	26	24	23	22	21	19	18	17	16	14
6'1"	1.8	33	32	30	29	28	26	25	24	22	21	20	18	17	16	15
6'0"	1.8	34	33	31	30	29	27	26	24	23	22	20	19	18	16	15
5'11"	1.8	35	33	32	31	30	28	26	25	24	22	21	20	18	17	15
5'10"	1.7	36	34	33	32	31	29	27	26	24	23	22	20	19	17	16
5'9"	1.7	37	35	34	33	32	30	28	27	25	24	22	21	19	18	16
5'7"	1.7	39	38	36	35	34	32	30	28	27	25	23	22	20	19	17
5'6"	1.6	40	39	37	36	35	33	31	29	27	26	24	23	21	19	18
5'5"	1.6	42	40	38	37	36	34	32	30	28	27	25	23	22	20	18
5'4"	1.6	43	41	39	38	37	35	33	31	29	27	26	24	22	21	19
5'3"	1.6	44	43	41	39	38	36	34	32	30	28	27	25	23	21	19
5'2"	1.5	46	44	42	40	39	37	35	33	31	29	27	26	24	22	20
5'1"	1.5	47	46	43	42	40	38	36	34	32	30	28	26	25	23	20
5'0"	1.5	49	47	45	43	41	39	37	35	33	31	29	27	25	23	21
4'11"	1.5	51	49	47	44	42	40	38	36	34	32	30	28	26	24	22
4'10"	1.4	52	50	48	46	44	42	40	38	36	33	31	29	27	25	23
Weight (lbs)		250	240	230	220	210	200	190	180	170	160	150	140	130	120	110

Figure 2.1 Calculator for BMI (kg/m^2).

3 ANTI-OBESITY AGENTS

Historical developments

Two drugs are presently approved for the treatment of obesity in the UK: orlistat (introduced 1998) and sibutramine (2001). These agents should be used in conjunction with lifestyle measures, especially a calorie-reduced diet.

Anti-obesity agents are not specifically indicated for the treatment of type 2 diabetes, but studies have consistently shown that improved weight loss in overweight and obese type 2 diabetes is associated with improved glycaemic control.

Bariatric surgery is receiving increased use to treat obesity, and an adjustable gastric band (LAP-BAND, Allergan) has received a licence amendment (2009) for control and remission of type 2 diabetes in selected obese patients.

Orlistat

Orlistat *(Xenical)* is a lipase inhibitor that acts in the GI tract to reduce fat digestion. It is derived from a lipase inhibitor produced by *Streptomyces toxytricini.* In 2009 orlistat became available as a non-prescription pharmacist-supplied medicine *(Alli)* in the UK.

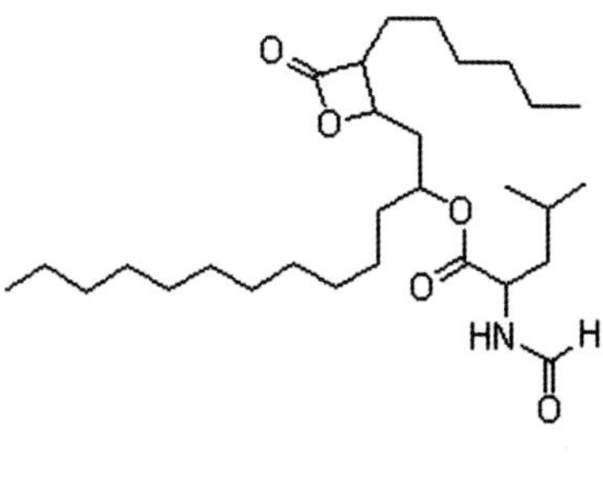

Figure 3.1 Structure of orlistat.

Table 3.1 Pharmacokinetics of orlistat	
Absorption	Absorption nominal (acts within GI tract)
Distribution	Almost all within GI tract. Plasma conc <10 ng/mL (0.02 μmol/L) about 42% of which is very weakly active metabolites. No significant systemic activity identified Systemic concentration too low for PK analysis
Metabolism	Metabolised in wall of GI tract to two metabolites with very weak activity (<1000 fold of active drug)
Elimination	Almost all eliminated in faeces, 83% unchanged. Trivial amounts of metabolites in plasma are eliminated in urine.

Mode of action

- Long-acting inhibitor of GI lipases
- Acts within the lumen of the alimentary tract to covalently bind at the active 'serine' site on the lipases
- This slows the digestion of dietary fats
- Orlistat can decrease the amount of fat absorbed by up to ~30%

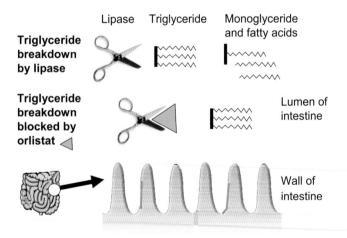

Figure 3.2 Mode of action of orlistat, an intestinal lipase inhibitor.

Indications

- Adjunct to lifestyle changes to assist reduction in adiposity for obese (BMI >30 kg/m^2) adults, or overweight (BMI ≥28 kg/m^2) patients with associated risk factors such as type 2 diabetes, hypertension or hypercholesterolaemia
- Orlistat can be used in overweight/obese type 2 diabetes patients treated with antidiabetic agents (caution with metformin, not recommended with acarbose)

Dose

- P medicine is 60 mg capsules
    - suggested dose is 60 mg tds with meals for up to 6 months
- POM is 120 mg capsules.
    - usual prescribed dose is 120 mg with meals up to three times daily for up to 2 yrs

Before starting therapy

- Patient should have achieved >2.5 kg weight loss over previous month with lifestyle changes, particularly a calorie-reduced diet.

Starting therapy

- Start with 120 mg immediately before, with, or up to 1hr after a main meal.
- Titrate up by adding further doses of 120 mg with other meals, up to a maximum of 360 mg/day. Appreciate possible GI side effects from the start.
- Continue to advise a calorie-reduced diet during use of orlistat, and advise a reduction in fat content.

Efficacy

- Orlistat with a calorie-reduced diet produced average weight loss of about 5-6 kg (compared with 3-4 kg on diet only) over 1 year in obese type 2 patients
- HbA1c was reduced by ~ 0.5% (~5 mmol/mol) in type 2 diabetes patients with a starting HbA1c >8% (>64 mmol/mol)
- Small reductions in circulating triglycerides and LDLc are often observed

Contra-indications

- Chronic malabsorption diseases
- Cholestasis
- Breast feeding and pregnancy are regarded as contra-indications although no adverse effects are known
- Known previous hypersensitivity to drug or excipients

Adverse effects

- Loose oily stools, faecal urgency and spotting
- Occasionally faecal incontinence, flatulence and abdominal discomfort

Precautions

- Side effects can be minimised by reducing the fat content of the diet
- Orlistat can potentially reduce absorption of fat-soluble vitamins (A, D, E, K, β-carotene). A once-daily multivitamin supplement may be helpful, taken at least 2 hours apart from orlistat
- Advise on possible failure of oral contraception and suggest additional contraception
- Caution is recommended if used in the elderly, although there is no evidence relating to hepatic or renal disease
- Orlistat is not licensed for use in children but the BNF indicates use in children >12 years if initiated by a specialist.

- Caution with ciclosporin, warfarin and antiepileptic agents
- Not recommended to use with acarbose, and caution with metformin
- If a meal is missed or contains no fat, omit the dose of orlistat
- Compliance is often an issue with weight-lowering therapy and continued support is important

Discontinue therapy

- Discontinue if weight loss is
    - < 5% loss of initial body weight at 3 months, or
    - < 10% loss of initial body weight at 6 months
- These levels of weight loss are not realistic for many patients, but therapy may still be beneficial and continued
- Maximum treatment period 2 years

Sibutramine

Sibutramine *(Reductil)* is a centrally acting satiety-inducing agent that reduces meal size

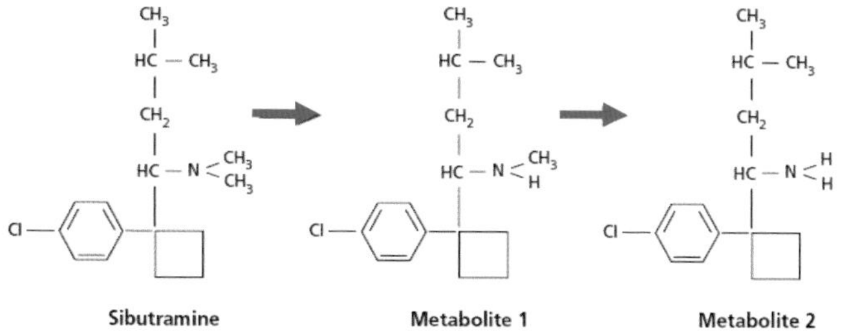

Figure 3.3 Structure of sibutramine and its two active metabolites, M1 (secondary amine) and M2 (primary amine)

Mode of action

- Serotonin (5-hydroxytryptamine) and noradrenaline re-uptake inhibitor (SNRI)
- Acts centrally to induce satiety effect

Table 3.2 Pharmacokinetics of sibutramine

Absorption	Well absorbed (~77%), Tmax ~1hr
Distribution	Sibutramine and metabolites >90% plasma protein bound
Metabolism	Rapidly metabolised mainly by CYP3A4 in the liver to the secondary (M1) and primary (M2) amine metabolites that are largely responsible for the drug's activity. Metabolite plasma Tmax ~3h, t½ 14-16hr
Elimination	Bile for sibutramine and active metabolites Mostly urine for inactive metabolites

- Most of its activity mediated through its secondary and primary amine metabolites.
- These metabolites increase the duration of serotonin and noradrenaline in the synaptic cleft.
- Dopamine re-uptake is marginally reduced, but there is no stimulatory effect on monoamine release.
- Sibutramine and its metabolites also act centrally to increase thermogenic energy expenditure via sympathetic pathways, and by direct peripheral metabolic effects.

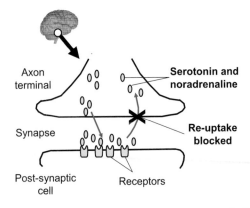

Figure 3.4 Mode of action of sibutramine.
This is a serotonin and noradrenaline re-uptake inhibitor (SNRI) that increases the duration of these transmitters in the synaptic cleft.

Indications

- Adjunct to lifestyle changes to assist reduction in adiposity for obese (BMI >30 kg/m^2) individuals, or overweight (BMI ≥27 kg/m^2) patients with associated risk factors such as type 2 diabetes or hypercholesterolaemia
- Sibutramine can be used in overweight/obese type 2 diabetes patients treated with antidiabetic agents

Dose

- Dose 10 or 15 mg od

Before starting therapy

- Patients should have made one or more serious attempts to lose weight by lifestyle changes for ≥ 3 months, but failed to achieve weight loss of 5%

Starting therapy

- Start with 10 mg od in the morning.
- Titrate up by to 15 mg od if weight loss <2 kg at 1 month.
- Continue to advise a calorie-reduced diet during use of sibutramine

Efficacy

- In overweight and obese type 2 diabetic patients, sibutramine produced average weight loss of about 2-4 kg more than diet only over 1 year
- HbA1c was reduced by ~ 0.5% (~5 mmol/mol) in type 2 diabetes patients and some patients reduced their dose of antidiabetic medication (metformin or insulin)
- Small reductions in circulating triglycerides and LDLc, and increased HDLc are sometimes observed

Contra-indications

- Inadequately controlled hypertension
- History of serious eating disorders (eg. anorexia nervosa)

- Psychiatric illness and Tourette's syndrome
- History of cardiovascular disease: coronary artery disease, congestive heart failure, peripheral vascular disease, stroke, TIA, arrhythmia or tachycardia
- Severe hepatic or renal impairment
- Hyperthyroidism, phaeochromocytoma
- Benign prostatic hyperplasia
- Narrow angle glaucoma
- Pregnancy and breast feeding
- Children <18 years or very elderly due to lack of information
- Known previous hypersensitivity to drug or excipients

Adverse effects
- Increased blood pressure and heart rate
- Occasionally anorexia, dry mouth, constipation, insomnia or asthenia

Monitoring
- Monitor blood pressure and heart rate frequently eg. every 2 weeks for first 3 months when changes are most likely

Precautions
- Potential drug interactions with inhibitors (eg. ketoconazole, erythromycin) or inducers (eg. rifampicin, phenytoin, carbamazepine, phenobarbital, dexamethasone) of CYP3A4, highly plasma protein bound drugs or recent use of centrally acting drugs (eg. antidepressants)
- Compliance is often an issue with weight-lowering therapy and continued support is important

Discontinue therapy
- Discontinue if 15 mg od does not produce weight loss of
  ≥ 2 kg at 1 month, or
  $\geq 5\%$ of initial body weight at 3 months, or
  ≥ 3 kg weight regain from previous weight loss
- Maximum treatment period 1 year.

4 TARGETS, GUIDELINES AND MONITORING

Aims and importance of glycaemic control

The aims of diabetes therapies are to
* Preserve life
* Alleviate symptoms
* Improve glycaemic control
* Prevent or reduce complications

Treatment of hyperglycaemia should be
* Early
* Effective
* Individualised

Ideally, treatment should
* Reinstate glycaemic control as near to normal as safely possible and practical, consistent with the circumstances of the individual.

Preferably, treatment should at least partially
* Correct underlying endocrine pathophysiological defects (insulin resistance, β-cell dysfunction and α-cell dysfunction)
* Address the metabolic sequelae (glucotoxicity and lipotoxicity)
* Provide durable control and containment of complications

Improved glycaemic control has been shown to:
* Delay or prevent the onset and reduce the severity of microvascular complications
  - these benefits continue to accrue until normoglycaemia is achieved
* Reduce the long-term risk of macrovascular complications
  - this may be associated with improvements in insulin resistance and the metabolic syndrome

Early intervention is paramount because
- Most patients have already had 'undiagnosed' diabetes for a long time (estimated to be about 10 years for many type 2 patients) before diagnosis
- The undiagnosed period of diabetes is associated with development of complications in 25-50% of patients by the time of diagnosis
- Deferred intervention increases the risk and severity of complications later in life, even if control is latterly improved ('glycaemic memory')

Careful assessment at each stage is crucial because
- Diabetes is life-long
- Most therapies will be for years or decades (or life-long for insulin treatment of type 1 diabetes)
- Treatments can have deferred effects on patient well-being decades into the future
- Inappropriate or over-intensive therapy can cause hypoglycaemia (excessively low blood glucose)
- Hypoglycaemia
  - impairs cognitive function,
  - seriously detracts from quality of life
  - can cause fatal glucopenic coma if unrecognised or untreated
  - incurs increased susceptibility to fatality after an MI
- Most patients will suffer co-morbidity which will impinge on the suitability of treatments
- Most patients will receive multiple medications with increased risk of interactions

Individualised and flexible regimens are necessary because
- Diabetes is heterogeneous and highly variable in its presentation and natural history
- Treatment needs to be adapted to the daily routine of the individual, to take account of different and changing patient circumstances, accommodate co-morbidities and other medications, be compatible with particular demands of occupations or patients living alone

Patient empowerment is required because
- Effective management depends upon the participation of the patient
  - to be able to take informed decisions
  - to take personal responsibility for day-to-day aspects of their own management including lifestyle measures, adjustments to the timing and dose of medications,
  - to maintain vigilance to watch for clinical problems

Special consideration of vulnerable individuals
- Elderly
- Children
- Neglectful living
- Unstable disease
- Advanced complications

Treatment algorithms

Drug treatments for diabetes should always be considered as adjuncts to lifestyle measures, and these measures should be reinforced throughout.

Type 1 diabetes
Initiate immediate insulin therapy immediately along with lifestyle measures (discussed in chapter 13).

After initial stabilisation, treatment may require adjustment periodically, usually to minimise daily fluctuations in glycaemia.

Type 2 diabetes
Since type 2 diabetes is progressive, it requires frequent up-titration or addition of extra therapies along with lifestyle measures.

Glucose-lowering therapies

To enable the management of hyperglycaemia to be tailored to the individual, many different types of antidiabetic medications are available to target hyperglycaemia in different ways .

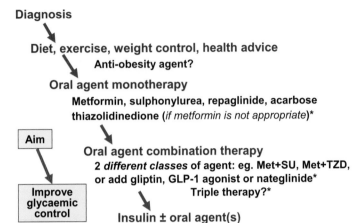

Diagnosis

Diet, exercise, weight control, health advice
        Anti-obesity agent?

        Oral agent monotherapy
        Metformin, sulphonylurea, repaglinide, acarbose
        thiazolidinedione (*if metformin is not appropriate*)*

Aim

        Oral agent combination therapy
        2 *different classes* of agent: eg. Met+SU, Met+TZD,
        or add gliptin, GLP-1 agonist or nateglinide*
                        Triple therapy?*

Improve glycaemic control

        Insulin ± oral agent(s)

* Licence restrictions, see text

Figure 4.1 Generalised algorithm for the treatment of hyperglycaemia in type 2 diabetes.

Table 4.1 Summary of glucose-lowering drugs and their main modes of action

Class with examples	Main mode of glucose-lowering	Main cellular mechanisms
ORAL		
Biguanide Metformin	Counter insulin resistance (especially decrease hepatic glucose output)	Enhance several insulin dependent and independent actions
Sulphonylureas Glimepiride Gliclazide Glibenclamide[a] Glipizide	Stimulate insulin secretion (typically 6-24 hours	Direct effect on pancreatic β-cells, bind to SUR1 receptors which closes K+ATP channels.

Most guidelines suggest the desirable targets for glycaemic control should be HbA1c ≤6.5-7.5% (48-59 mmol/mol). However, it is increasingly acknowledged that the lower part of this range may be impractical, unrealistic and undesirable for some patients. Thus most guidelines now recognise the importance of treatment that is individualised to the circumstances of the patient.

Progressive nature of type 2 diabetes

When type 2 diabetes is diagnosed insulin resistance is usually well established and changes little thereafter. Advancement of the disease, with continued escalation of hyperglycaemia, is largely due to the progressive loss of β-cell function.

If adequate control is not achieved or not maintained, this is customarily addressed by titrating up drug doses and increasing the number of antidiabetic therapies. Do not delay this process: extended periods of poor control make reinstatement of good control more difficult and increase risk of complications.

Poor control early after diagnosis can also predispose to complications much later in the natural history of the disease, even when control is subsequently improved (glycaemic memory or legacy effect).

Table 4.3   Typical sequence of therapies for type 2 diabetes

Lifestyle advice	Reinforced at all stages
Monotherapy	At least one oral agent is tried first (if patient is severely hyperglycaemic and symptomatic, insulin may be preferred)
Combination of two agents	Addition of a second, *differently acting* oral agent and/or injected GLP-1 agonist
Triple therapy	Use of three differently acting agents other than insulin
Insulin +/- other agent(s)	Typically introduce basal insulin and continue metformin or another oral agent. Intensify insulin therapy with a more complex regimen in more severely affected patients

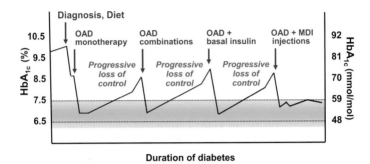

Figure 4.2   Typical long-term scenario for management of hyperglycaemia in type 2 diabetes.
As the disease progresses each therapy is eventually unable to maintain control and additional therapies are required.

Guidelines

In the UK, prescribers are encouraged to follow the NICE guidelines, currently guideline 87 (published May 2009) for the treatment of type 2 diabetes.

NICE guideline 87 recognises the need for flexibility and individualisation of treatment to address the varied and progressive difficulty of sustaining glycaemic control, eg. initially HbA1c <6.5% (48 mmol/mol) if appropriate and safe, but in more advanced stages of the disease <7.5% (59 mmol/mol) may be a more realistic target.

NICE guideline 87 proposes a preferred sequence in which individual agents should normally be considered.

Most guidelines also recognise
* Structured education for all newly diagnosed patients and/or carers, then reinforcement and review on an annual basis.
* Blood pressure target of <140/80 mmHg (<130/80 mmHg if renal, eye or cerebrovascular disease)
* Simvastatin 40 mg, or equivalent, in all type 2 diabetes aged >40 years, irrespective of CV disease (aim TC < 4 mmol/L; LDLc <2 mmol/L)

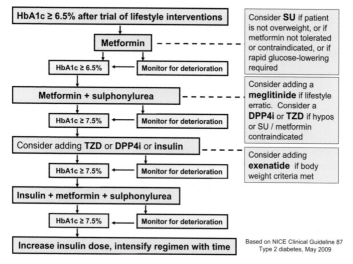

Figure 4.3 A simplified version of the NICE guideline 87 for the treatment of hyperglycaemia.

Reimbursement targets

- Reimbursements for diabetes treatment in general practice (2009/2010) in the UK are based on the percentage of patients with diabetes in whom the last HbA1c in the past 15 months was below specified targets.

Table 4.4 Indicators of diabetes control used for reimbursement in general practice in the UK (# 23, 24, 25)

HbA1c	Points	Threshold
≤ 7%	17	40-50%
≤ 8%	8	40-70%
≤ 9%	10	40-90%

Starting glucose-lowering therapy

- The aim of therapy is to achieve optimum glucose control with the lowest effective amount of drug(s) administered.
- When adding therapies they should have a different mechanism of action

Table 4.5 General principles to apply when starting glucose-lowering therapy

Drug selection	Patient circumstances
	    Pathophysiological status
	    Lifestyle
	    Co-morbidities
	    Concurrent medications
	    Individualised glycaemic target
	Contraindications and cautions

Dose – start low	Once daily (usually with breakfast) if using an intermediate or long-acting agent
	or
	Twice daily (usually with breakfast and mid-day/early evening meal) if using a short-acting agent
	Patient to monitor blood glucose:
	    before breakfast and 1-2 h after main meal
	or
	    at least 2 days/wk during first 1-2 wks

Dose – increase	If target control or significant decrease in blood glucose not achieved by 2-4 wks increase dosage Most drugs are titrated at 1-2 wk intervals Some agents (eg. TZDs) have a slow onset of efficacy, and may be titrated at 4-8 wk intervals
Ongoing glucose monitoring	As dosage increases consider use of intermediate or long-acting drugs in divided doses Increase vigilance: for hypoglycaemia (interprandial and nocturnal) and drug interactions
If glycaemic control is not improved	If increased dosage does not improve glycaemic control adequately over 4 wks: return to previous dosage level
If glycaemic control is unsatisfactory with maximum effective dosage	With monotherapy: add a 2nd agent* or commence insulin (± oral agent) With dual combination therapy - add a 3rd agent* or commence insulin (± oral agents)

* Add agent with a different cellular mode of action. May involve starting an injectable drug, eg. GLP-1 agonist or insulin.

Changing and stopping drug therapy in type 2 diabetes

Temporarily stop oral therapy and add insulin if:
- Change in lifestyle and daily routine
- Intercurrent illness
- Investigations (eg. intravenous pyelography, angiography)
- Changes in co-morbidities especially CV or other events
- Changes in drugs for co-morbidities
- Elective surgery
- Chronic debilitating illness
- Pregnancy
- Malnutrition

Do not stop insulin completely because it is needed for purposes other than glucose control, including, growth, cellular differentiation and the control of other aspects of nutrient metabolism.

If no meals are taken, then omit bolus (rapid/short-acting) doses of insulin and reduce the basal (intermediate/long-acting) insulin as required.

Glucose monitoring

HbA1c (glycated haemoglobin)
- The proportion of haemoglobin with glucose attached (slow non-enzymatic reaction)
- Indicates long-term glycaemic control during the previous 6-8 wks
- Should be checked at least every 6 months at patient reviews
- Blood can be taken at any time
- Reference range for non-diabetic individuals typically 4-6 % (20-42 mmol/mol)
- Inappropriate measure in patients with haemoglobinopathies or other significant disturbances of red blood cells
- Does not indicate daily fluctuations in blood glucose control

A comparison of units for glucose and HbA1c measurements is given in Chapter 15.

Fructosamine
- The amount of serum protein with sugar attached (slow non-enzymatic reaction, main protein is albumin)
- Indicates medium-term glycaemic control during previous 2-3 wks
- Not widely used in routine clinical practice
- Blood can be taken at any time
- Reference range for non-diabetic individuals typically 200-300 μmol/L
- Inappropriate to measure fructosamine in patients with severe hepatic disease affecting albumin turnover

Plasma glucose
- Concentration of glucose, usually measured by a laboratory in venous plasma
- Standard measurement for diagnosis of diabetes:
      - random or 2h OGTT ≥11.1 mmol/L (200 mg/dL)
      - overnight fasted ≥7 mmol/L (126 mg/dL)
- Standard measurement for acute glycaemic assessment and drug dose titration
- Very sensitive to time of blood sample
- Reference range for non-diabetic individuals:
      - overnight fasted 4-6 mmol/L, (72-108 mg/dL)
      - 1h postprandial 5-10 mmol/L (90-180 mg/dL)

Capillary blood glucose
- Usually taken using finger-stick blood glucose meter
- Meters are usually calibrated to give a venous plasma equivalent value
- Mainstay for self-monitoring of blood glucose (SMBG) by patients
- Very helpful in recognising glycaemic fluctuations, normal daily self-management and reassurance, confirming and averting symptoms of hypoglycaemia, and drug dose adjustment
- Under stable conditions self-monitoring is suggested one day per week

5 METFORMIN

Historical developments

Metformin (*Glucophage*) is the only biguanide used in the UK, and it is the most widely prescribed oral antidiabetic therapy worldwide. Its discovery stems from the use of *Galega officinalis* (goat's rue or French lilac) as a traditional treatment for symptoms of diabetes in medieval Europe. *G. officinalis* is rich in the glucose-lowering substance guanidine from which metformin is derived. Metformin was introduced in the UK in the early 1960s. In 1998 the UKPDS reported that metformin improved microvascular and macrovascular outcomes in type 2 diabetes.

Metformin counters insulin resistance and exerts beneficial anti-atherothrombotic effects that are independent of blood glucose-lowering. Most guidelines presently recommend metformin as initial antidiabetic therapy for type 2 diabetes.

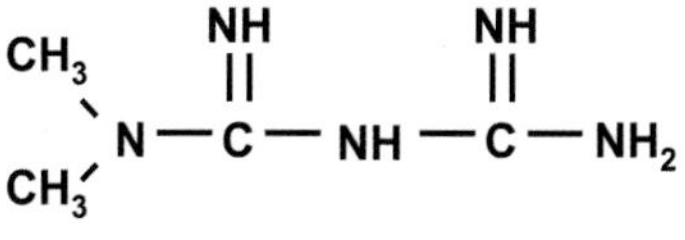

Figure 5.1 Structure of metformin.

Table 5.1 Pharmacokinetics of metformin	
Absorption	50-60% absorbed, this decreases at high doses Mainly from upper small intestine T_{max} 1-3 h (4-8h for prolonged release formulation)
Distribution	Distributes widely, negligible protein binding Plasma C_{max} ~1-2 μg/ml (10^{-5}M). Very high concentration in intestinal wall serves as drug reservoir. There are also high concentrations in kidney, liver and salivary glands
Metabolism	Not metabolised
Elimination	Urine ~ 100% $t\frac{1}{2}$ ~ 6h

41

Mode of action

- Counters insulin resistance by several insulin-dependent and insulin-independent mechanisms
- Main glucose-lowering effect appears to be a decrease in hepatic glucose production
- Modest increase in peripheral glucose uptake, storage and utilisation
- Increase in glucose turnover between the intestine and liver.

Table 5.2 Antihyperglycaemic actions of metformin

	Insulin-dependent	Insulin-independent
Liver	↓ Gluconeogenesis ↓ Glucagon action ↓ Glycogenolysis ↓ G-6-Pase	↓ Gluconeogenesis ↓ Lactate extraction
Muscle	↑ Glucose uptake ↑ Glycogenesis ↑ Glucose oxidation ↑ GLUT4 translocation	↓ FA oxidation
Gut		↑ Anaerobic glycolysis ↓ Respiratory chain site 1 ↑ Glucose turnover

↑ increase; ↓ decrease

Key features

- Reduces effect of insulin resistance
- Requires presence of some insulin for glucose-lowering efficacy
- Does not stimulate insulin secretion
- Does not cause overt hypoglycaemia when used as monotherapy
- Does not cause weight gain: may facilitate small weight reduction
- Improves several components of 'metabolic syndrome' through which it can reduce cardiovascular risk independently of glucose control

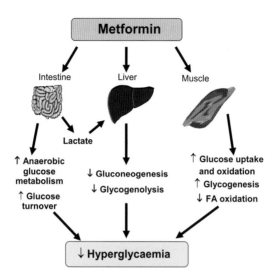

Figure 5.2 Mode of action of metformin. ↑ *increase;* ↓ *decrease*

Table 5.3 Effects of metformin on the cardiovascular risk indicators of 'metabolic syndrome'

	Effects of metformin
Insulin resistance	Decrease, by insulin-dependent and insulin-independent mechanisms
Hyperinsulinaemia	Reduce fasting insulin and proinsulin
Abdominal obesity	Stabilise or reduce visceral fat: may facilitate overall small weight reduction
Hyperglycaemia	Improve glycaemic control in type 2 diabetes and IGT
Dyslipidaemia	Modest benefits: can ↓ TG and ↓ LDL-c in hyperlipidaemic patients; small ↑ HDL-c
Raised blood pressure	No change or slight ↓ BP associated with weight loss
Coagulation status	Decrease thrombotic risk: ↓ PAI-1, ↓ fibrinogen and ↓ platelet aggregation
Pro-inflammatory markers	Decrease some markers eg. CRP
Atherosclerosis	Decrease some markers eg. adhesion molecules and monocyte differentiation Decrease MI events and increase survival in UKPDS

↑ increase; ↓ decrease

Indications

Type 2 diabetes

- In adults who are inadequately controlled by lifestyle measures alone or with other antidiabetic agents
- Often preferred for overweight and obese patients
- Monotherapy or in combination with any other class of glucose-lowering agents including insulin
- In children from 10 yrs of age and adolescents with appropriate caution

Dose

- Metformin should be taken immediately before or with main meals

Table 5.4 Dosage strengths and formulations of metformin

Dosage	500 mg, 750 mg, 850 mg and 1000 mg od, bd or tds	
Formulations	500 mg	- tablet (IR and SR), - sachet, - liquid (500 mg/mL)
	750 mg	- tablet (SR)
	850 mg	- tablet (IR)
	1000 mg	- tablet (IR and SR), - sachet

Maximum dose mg/day	Recommended: 2000-2550 mg
	Licensed: 3000 mg IR
	                   (2000 mg in children and adolescents)
	                   2000 mg SR	

IR = immediate (standard) release
SR= slow (sustained) release

Starting therapy

- Newly diagnosed: trial of lifestyle measures first
- Check for contra-indications (especially renal)
- Introduce at low dose (500 mg or 850 mg od) at breakfast or other main meal
- Monitor fasting plasma glucose
- Up-titrate dose, 1 tablet at a time, every 1-2 weeks
- Always take with meals
- Use of SR formulation may reduce or avoid GI intolerance
- Increase dosage until desired glycaemic control achieved
- If a titration step does not improve glycaemic control or causes GI intolerance, return to previous dose, try re-titration later, and consider additional treatment if unable to achieve adequate glycaemic control.

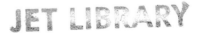

Combination therapy

- Metformin can be added when monotherapy with another agent, including insulin, does not achieve or sustain adequate glycaemic control
- Other agents can be added when metformin monotherapy is inadequate
- Metformin can be used to reduce insulin dose
- ~5-10% of patients per year do not sustain glycaemic control with metformin and require additional therapy

Table 5.5 Efficacy of metformin	
↓ HbA1c	~1-2% (~11-22 mmol/mol) if starting HbA1c >8% (>64 mmol/mol).
↓ FPG	1-4 mmol/L (18-72 mg/dL)
Lipids	↓ TG, ↓ TC and ↓ FFA in some dyslipidaemic states
Other	Body weight typically unchanged Basal insulin concentrations unchanged or slightly reduced Overt hypoglycaemia unlikely as monotherapy

↑ increase; ↓ decrease

Contra-indications

Renal dysfunction or disease

Eg. If serum creatinine >130 μmol/L or creatinine clearance <60 mL/min

NICE has suggested review metformin dose if serum creatinine >130 μmol/L or eGFR <45mL/min/1.73m^2 and caution with those at risk of a sudden deterioration in kidney function, and stop if serum creatinine >150 μmol/L or eGFR <30 mL/min/1.73m^2

Hypoxaemic conditions

Eg. cardiac insufficiency causing tissue hypoxia, recent MI, severe respiratory insufficiency, acute shock, septicaemia or severe infection

- ***History of lactic acidosis***
  Or other metabolic acidosis including diabetic ketoacidosis
- ***Significant liver disease***
- ***Pregnancy and breast feeding***
  Not recommended, but no adverse effects have been reported
- ***Hypersensitivity***
  Known previous hypersensitivity to metformin or excipients

Adverse effects

- ***Risk of lactic acidosis***
  This is usually due to unrecognised onset of renal contra-indication. Lactic acidosis occurs in ~0.03/1000 patient years of treatment: ~50% of cases are fatal. Lactic acidosis is an emergency (Chapter 14)
- ***GI side effects***
  Diarrhoea and abdominal discomfort, nausea and metallic taste are experienced by about 20% of patients starting metformin IR. These are usually transient and remit with time, or with re-titration and taking with meals, or substitution with SR. However about 5% of patients do not tolerate any metformin
- ***B12 malabsorption***
  Vitamin B12 absorption reduced. This is rarely sufficient to precipitate overt anaemia
  Reduced folate absorption has been reported
- ***Hypoglycaemia***
  Can occur when metformin is used in combination with an insulin releasing agent or insulin

Precautions

- Monitor for contra-indicationss
- Check serum creatinine at least annually, more frequently if already high or rising steadily.
- Potential drug interaction with cimetidine (compete for renal clearance)
- Avoid significant intake of alcohol

- Suggest check haemoglobin, especially if already low.
- Special caution in children, particularly aged 10-12 yrs
- In PCOS menstruation and ovulation can restart
- Caution is advised in pregnancy although use at this time has not been associated with adverse outcomes

Discontinue therapy

- If contra-indications develop
- Stop for elective use of contrast media investigations until normal renal function returns

6 SULPHONYLUREAS

Historical developments

Sulphonylureas were developed after observations that sulphonamide drugs could cause hypoglycaemia. Sulphonylureas were introduced in the UK in the late 1950s and for several decades were the most commonly used treatment for type 2 diabetes. Sulphonylureas act on the pancreas to stimulate insulin secretion by the islet β-cell.

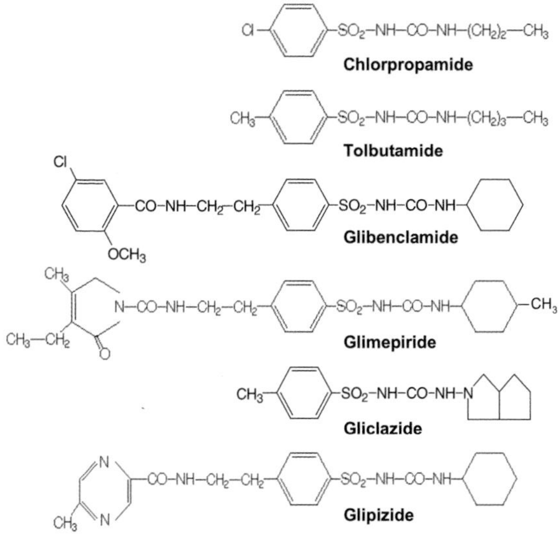

Figure 6.1   *Structure of sulphonylureas*

The structural differences between sulphonylureas alter the manner in which they bind to the SUR1 on the β-cell, which alters their duration of action

* 1st generation sulphonylureas exhibit low affinity binding and are generally given in larger doses (eg tolbutamide, chlorpropamide)

- Chlorpropamide is no longer recommended for new patients due to a long half life and side effects
- 2nd generation sulphonylureas exhibit higher binding affinity for SUR1 and are given in lower doses (eg. glibenclamide, glipizide, gliclazide and glimepiride)
- Sulphonylureas are almost completely absorbed from the intestine
- Almost all sulphonylureas reach T_{max} in 2-4 hrs and they are highly (>85%) protein bound
- The different structures of sulphonylureas considerably alter their metabolism, the activity of metabolites and elimination

Table 6.1 Pharmacokinetics of sulphonylureas					
Drug	**Daily dose mg**	**Duration of action h**	**Metabolite activity**	**Elimination**	
				Time t½ h	**Route***
1st generation					
Tolbutamide	500-2000	6-12	Inactive	4-7 (28)	Urine ~100%
Chlorpropamide	100-500	24-50	Active	24-50	Urine >90%
2nd generation					
Glibenclamide	2.5-15	18-24	Active	10-20 (>24)	Bile >50%
Gliclazide	40-320	12-20	Inactive	6-14 (20)	Urine ~65%
Gliclazide MR	30-120	~24	Inactive	~17	Urine ~65%
Glimepiride	1-6	18-24	Active	5-9 (~24)	Urine ~60%
Glipizide	2.5-15	6-16	Inactive	2-7	Urine ~70%

Gliclazide MR (Diamicron MR) is a modified release formulation given at a lower dosage that produces a greater duration of action
* (includes metabolites)

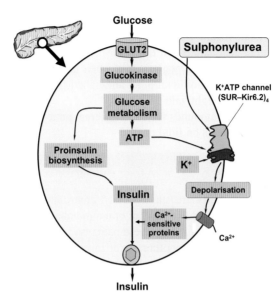

Figure 6.2   Mode of action of sulphonylureas to stimulate insulin secretion by pancreatic β-cells

Mode of action

- Direct action on pancreatic β-cells to stimulate insulin secretion
- Bind to sulphonylurea receptor SUR1:
  this closes K^+ATP channels which reduces K^+ efflux, which depolarises the membrane and opens voltage- dependent Ca^{2+} channels; this in turn increases intracellular Ca^{2+} which activates Ca^{2+}-dependent proteins that regulate insulin release
- Sulphonylureas can initiate insulin secretion at low glucose concentrations (hence risk of hypoglycaemia)
- Some sulphonylureas may have weak extra-pancreatic effects to reduce hepatic glucose output and potentiate peripheral glucose uptake, but it is uncertain whether such effects are clinically significant
- Sulphonylureas may transiently reduce glucagon release

Key features

- Stimulate insulin release
- Require adequate β-cell function
- Can cause overt hypoglycaemia when used as monotherapy and in combination with other antidiabetic agents
- May cause weight gain
- Variety of compounds suited to different patient groups
- Minimal effects on lipid profile

Indications

Type 2 diabetes
- In adults who are inadequately controlled by lifestyle measures alone or with other oral antidiabetic agents
- Often preferred for non-obese patients
- Can be used as monotherapy or in combination with any other class of glucose-lowering agent including insulin, but not normally used with a meglitinide as this combination gives no added benefit due to similar cellular mode of action

Dose

- Doses of sulphonylureas vary according to their binding affinity for SUR1 and their duration of action

Starting therapy

- Newly diagnosed: trial of lifestyle measures first
- Check for contraindications
- Select on basis of:
    - duration of action compatible with lifestyle,
    - mode of metabolism and elimination compatible with hepatic and renal status and other medications
- Caution with long-acting agents in the elderly
- Introduce at low dose once daily, usually with breakfast
- Monitor fasting plasma glucose
- Up-titrate dose at ~2 week intervals
- Short/intermediate-acting (tolbutamide, gliclazide, glipizide) can be given in divided doses with meals

Table 6.2 Sulphonylurea tablet strengths and doses

Drug	Tablet strength mg	Start dose mg/d	Max dose mg/day	Caution
Tolbutamide *All generic*	500	500	2000	Renal
Chlorpropamide** *All generic*	100, 250	100	500	Renal, elderly
Glibenclamide *Euglucon*	2.5, 5*	2.5	15	Renal, hepatic, elderly
Gliclazide *Diamicron*	80*	40	320	Renal, hepatic
Gliclazide MR *Diamicron MR*	30*	30	120	Renal, hepatic
Glimepiride *Amaryl*	1*,2*,3*,4*	1	4***	Renal, hepatic
Glipizide *Glibenese Minodiab*	2.5, 5*	2.5	20	Renal

*   Tablets scored
**   No longer recommended for new patients
***   Max dose exceptionally 6mg/day

- Longer acting sulphonylureas (glibenclamide, glimepiride, gliclazide MR) usually once daily, but can be given twice daily provided consideration is given to potential nocturnal hypoglycaemia (chlorpropamide is once daily, but not for new patients)
- Always take with meals
- Risk of hypoglycaemia (harmonise with meals and exercise, advise on symptoms of hypoglycaemia and response)
     - suggest self monitoring of blood glucose if possible
- If patient experiences hypoglycaemia:
     - reduce one dosage level
     - consider adding small dose of differently acting antidiabetic agent
     - consider switching to shorter-acting secretagogue or alternative type of insulin releasing agent (eg. gliptin or GLP-1 agonist)

- Maximum effect is usually achieved at about half the maximum recommended dose
- If dose titration produces no benefit return to previous dose
    - consider starting combination therapy
- If starting or withdrawing any potentially interacting therapy check glycaemic control and adjust dose if required

Combination therapy

- Sulphonyureas can be added when monotherapy with another agent (except meglitinide), does not achieve or sustain adequate glycaemic control
- Other agents with different cellular modes of action can be added when sulphonlyurea monotherapy is inadequate
- Sulphonylurea can be used with insulin in type 2 diabetes when there is adequate remaining β-cell function
- About 10% of patients per year do not sustain glycaemic control with a sulphonlyurea and require additional therapy

Table 6.3 Efficacy of sulphonylureas	
↓ HbA1c	~1-2% (~11-22 mmol/mol) if starting HbA1c >8% (>64 mmol/mol)
↓ FPG	2-4 mmol/L (18-72 mg/dL)
Other	Immediate onset of glucose-lowering efficacy Efficacy often reduces over 1-2 yrs

Contra-indications

- *Significant renal disease*

    For sulphonylureas that are excreted mainly in the urine, notably chlorpropamide (not for new patients)

- *Significant hepatic disease*

    For sulphonylureas that are metabolised by the liver, eg. glibenclamide, gliclazide, glimepiride and glipizide

- *Serious cardiac conditions*

    Including recent MI, may require reconsideration of 2nd generation sulphonylureas with a benzamido moiety, eg. glibenclamide, glimepiride, glipizide, since these drugs may interact with SUR2A/B on cardiac and vascular smooth muscle

- ***Pregnancy and breast feeding***

  Not recommended, but no adverse effects have been reported

- ***Hypersensitivity***

  Known previous hypersensitivity (eg. skin rash) to sulphonylureas or excipients

- ***Porphyria***

  Sulphonylureas can cause acute aggravation

- ***Type 1 diabetes or previous ketosis***

Adverse effects

- ***Body weight gain***

  Typically ↑1-4kg, stabilising after ~6 months

- ***Hypoglycaemia***

  Is more likely with longer-acting sulphonylureas, in older patients and with longer duration of disease

  Is more likely in combination with other antidiabetic or anti-obesity drugs, or drugs that compete for plasma protein binding. Every year:

  ~20% of patients experience ≥1 episode of hypoglycaemia, mostly mild or moderate

  ~1% of patients experience an episode of severe hypoglycaemia: this is an emergency (Chapter 14)

  Incidence of fatal suphonylurea-induced hypoglycaemia is ~0.02/1000 patient years of treatment

Precautions

- Monitor glucose periodically after titration to ensure optimal control maintained
- Ensure patient can recognise and respond to symptoms of hypoglycaemia
- Avoid erratic eating habits
- Avoid significant intake of alcohol
- Check periodically for emergence of contraindications, especially renal or hepatic disease

Table 6.4 Potential drug interactions that could decrease the glucose-lowering effect of sulphonylureas

Glucocorticoids	Chronically antagonise insulin secretion and action
Nifedipine	Inhibits intracellular Ca^{2+} flux which inhibits insulin secretion
Octreotide	Decreases insulin secretion
Diazoxide	Opens K^+ATP channels
Diuretics	Various types of interaction

Table 6.5 Potential drug interactions that could increase the glucose-lowering effect of sulphonylureas

Intrinsic glucose-lowering activity	Other antidiabetic drugs Salicylates (high dose) Monoamine oxidase inhibitors Some quinolone antibacterials Alcohol
Displacement from plasma protein binding	Sulphonamides Warfarin Fibrates Phenylbutazone Salicylates (high dose)
Decreased hepatic metabolism	Warfarin Monoamine oxidase inhibitors Chloramphenicol Phenylbutazone and other NSAIDs Some antifungal agents
Decreased renal elimination	Salicylates (high dose) Probenecid Allopurinol

Beta adrenergic blockers can mask symptoms of hypoglycaemia and reduce counter-regulation

Discontinue therapy

- If contraindications develop
- If hypoglycaemia becomes an issue

7 MEGLITINIDES

Historical developments

Meglitindes were developed as short-acting prandial insulin releasers following the observation that meglitinide (the non-sulphonlyurea 'benzamido' region of glibenclamide) could stimulate insulin secretion. The two meglitinides, repaglinide and nateglinide were introduced in the UK in 1998 and 2001 respectively.

Repaglinide is a benzoic acid derivative and nateglinide is a structurally related derivative of the amino acid D-phenylalanine.

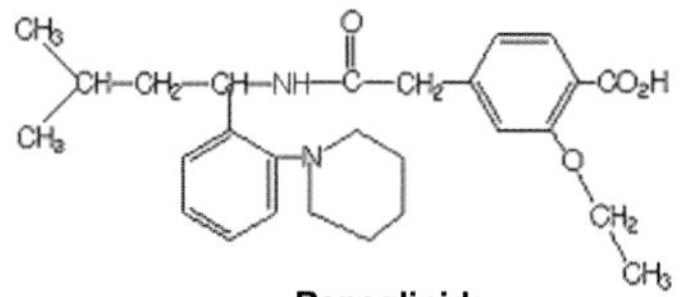

Repaglinide

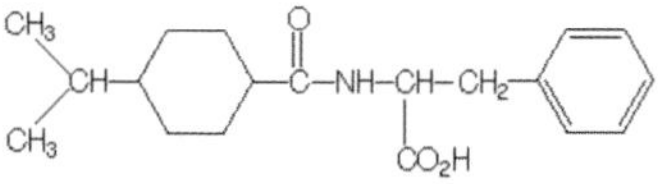

Nateglinide

Figure 7.1 Structure of repaglinide and nateglinide

Table 7.1 Pharmacokinetics of meglitinides

	Repaglinide	Nateglinide
Absorption	50-60% absorbed T_{max} <1 h	~70% absorbed. T_{max} <1 h
Distribution	>98% protein bound	>97% protein bound
Metabolism	Liver (100%) to inactive metabolites	Liver (>85%), mainly inactive metabolites, one minor metabolite is weakly active
Elimination	Bile ~90% t½ ~1.5 h	Urine ~80% t½ ~1.5 h

57

Mode of action

- Direct action on pancreatic β-cells to stimulate insulin secretion
- Faster onset of action and shorter duration of action than sulphonylureas
- Bind to benzamido site on sulphonylurea receptor SUR1. This site is separate from the sulphonylurea site on the same receptor, but elicits the same response

   Binding closes K⁺ATP channels which reduces K⁺ efflux. This depolarises the membrane and opens voltage dependent Ca^{2+} channels. Increased intracellular Ca^{2+} activates Ca^{2+}-dependent proteins that regulate insulin release

- Meglitinides can initiate insulin secretion at low glucose concentrations (thus risk of hypoglycaemia, but this is unlikely to be severe due to their short duration of action)

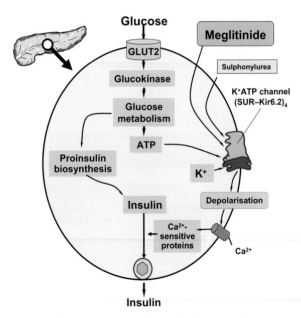

Figure 7.2   Mode of action of meglitinides to stimulate insulin secretion by pancreatic β-cells

Key features

- Stimulate insulin release
- Require adequate β-cell function
- Rapid but short duration of action, unlikely to precipitate severe hypoglycaemia when used as monotherapy (and if used appropriately with meals)
- Weight gain of 1-3 kg which stabilises in 1-3 months
- Minimal effects on lipid profile

Indications

Type 2 diabetes
- In adults who are inadequately controlled by lifestyle measures alone or with another oral antidiabetic agent.
- Often preferred for patients with erratic meal patterns or other susceptibility to hypoglycaemia eg. religious fasting such as during Ramadan
- More useful against postprandial (rather than basal) hyperglycaemia
- Mostly used in combination with metformin: no anticipated benefit with sulphonylureas; minimal anticipated benefit with gliptins or GLP-1 agonists as these already target prandial insulin secretion.

Dose

- Doses of meglitinides should be taken up to 30 min before meals or with meals.

Table 7.2 Meglitinide tablet strengths and doses

Drug	Tablet strength mg	Start dose mg/meal	Maximum dose mg/day	Caution
Repaglinide *Prandin*	0.5, 1, 2	0.5	16 (max 4 mg/meal)	Hepatic disease
Nateglinide *Starlix*	60, 120, 180	60	540 (max 180 mg/meal)	Hepatic disease

Starting therapy

- Newly diagnosed: trial of lifestyle measures first
- Check for contra-indications
- In the UK *repaglinide* can be used as first line or combination therapy, but *nateglinide* is only licensed as add-on therapy
- Select on basis of need for prandial insulin releaser
    - nateglinide tends to be slightly shorter acting than repaglinide.
- Introduce with main meal
- Up-titrate by increasing dose and/or adding treatment at other meals at ~1 week intervals
- Suggest self monitoring of blood glucose if possible.
- If patient experiences hypoglycaemia:
    - reduce one dosage level and/or omit/cut dosage at lesser meal
- If dose titration produces no benefit:
    - return to previous regimen
    - consider adding agent with different cellular mode of action
- If starting or withdrawing any potentially interacting therapy check glycaemic control and adjust regimen if required

Combination therapy

- A meglitinide can be added when adequate glycaemic control is not achieved or sustained by monotherapy with another agent that does not stimulate insulin secretion
- Other agents with different cellular modes of action can be added when repaglinide monotherapy is inadequate
- Meglitinides have been used off-label with insulin in type 2 diabetes when there is adequate remaining β-cell function

Table 7.3 Efficacy of meglitinides			
↓ HbA1c	Repaglinide Nateglinide	~0.5-1.5% ~0.5-1%	(>5-16 mmol/mol) (~5-11 mmol/mol)
↓ FPG	Repaglinide Nateglinide	1-3 mmol/L 1-2 mmol/L	(18-54 mg/dL) (18-36 mg/dL)
↓ PPG	Repaglinide Nateglinide	1-4 mmol/L 1-3 mmol/L	(18-72 mg/dL) (183- 54 mg/dL)

Contra-indications

* **Significant liver disease**

* **Pregnancy and breast feeding**
  Not recommended, but no adverse effects have been reported

* **Hypersensitivity**
  Known previous hypersensitivity (eg. skin rash) to meglitinides or excipients

* **Type 1 diabetes or previous ketosis**

Adverse effects

* **Body weight gain**
  May cause small gain in body weight

* **Hypoglycaemia**
  Low risk, not usually severe when used as monotherapy
  More likely in combination with other antidiabetic
  drugs or drugs that compete for plasma protein binding or interfere with hepatic metabolism

Precautions

Table 7.4 Potential drug interactions that could decrease the glucose-lowering effect of meglitinides	
Chronically antagonise insulin secretion and action	Glucocorticoids
Inducers of CYP3A5 and CYP2C9	Rifampicin, barbiturates and carbamazepine

- Monitor glucose periodically after titration to ensure optimal control maintained
- Ensure patient can recognise and respond to symptoms of hypoglycaemia
- Avoid significant intake of alcohol
- Check periodically for emergence of contra-indications, especially hepatic disease
- Serious cardiac conditions including recent MI may require reconsideration due to theoretical effect of interaction with SUR2A/B on cardiac and vascular smooth muscle.

Table 7.5 Potential drug interactions that could increase glucose-lowering effect of meglitinides

Intrinsic glucose-lowering activity	Other antidiabetic drugs
Displacement from plasma protein binding	Sulphonamides Warfarin Salicylates (high dose)
Decreased hepatic metabolism	Some antibacterial and antifungal agents Gemfibrozil, simvastatin Some oral contraceptive agents

Beta adrenergic blockers can mask symptoms of hypoglycaemia and reduce counter-regulation

Discontinue therapy

- If contra-indications develop
- If hypoglycaemia becomes an issue
- If side effects develop or risk of drug interactions

8 GLIPTINS

Historical developments

Gliptins are also known as DPP4 inhibitors since they act by inhibiting the action of the enzyme dipeptidyl peptidase-4. Development of gliptins followed the discovery that insulinotropic intestinal hormones (known as incretins) are rapidly degraded by DPP4. Inhibiting DPP4 increases the plasma half-life of incretin hormones which leads to increased insulin secretion. Two gliptins have been introduced in Europe: sitagliptin (*Januvia,* 2007), vildagliptin (*Galvus,* 2008).

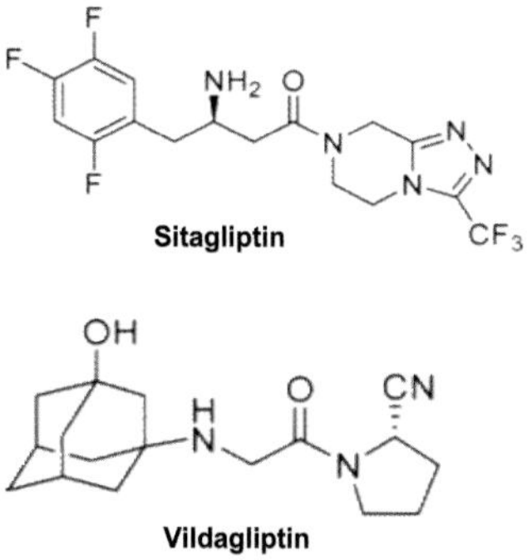

Sitagliptin

Vildagliptin

Figure 8.1 Structure of sitagliptin and vildagliptin.

Table 8.1 Pharmacokinetics of gliptins		
	Sitagliptin	**Vildagliptin**
Absorption	~87% absorbed T_{max} 1-4 h	~85% absorbed T_{max} ~1.7 h
Distribution	~38% protein bound	~9% protein bound
Metabolism	~20% metabolised (CYP3A4, CYP2C8), ~80% not metabolised	~69% metabolised (mostly kidney), mainly inactive metabolites
Elimination	~79% urine unchanged $t\frac{1}{2}$ ~12.4 h	~85% urine $t\frac{1}{2}$ 2-3 h

Mode of action

- Inhibits the activity of the enzyme DPP4 in the circulation.
    - DPP4 rapidly degrades the insulinotropic incretin hormones GLP-1 and GIP
    - thus, DPP4 inhibition enhances the levels of incretin hormones
    - incretins enhance glucose-induced insulin secretion
- By enhancing the effects of the incretin hormones, gliptins increase glucose-induced insulin secretion by the pancreatic β-cells, ie. they predominantly enhance prandial insulin secretion

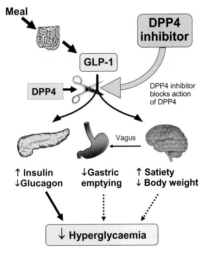

Figure 8.2   Mode of action of gliptins.
Via inhibition of the enzyme DPP4, gliptins cause an increase in circulating levels of the incretins GLP-1 and GIP which increase glucose-induced insulin secretion by pancreatic β-cells

- Note, whereas sulphonylureas and meglitinides act via K^+ATP channels and can initiate insulin secretion at low glucose concentrations, incretins (and gliptins via incretins) enhance glucose-induced insulin secretion but do not themselves initiate insulin secretion, ie. gliptins do not increase insulin secretion at low glucose concentrations

- Gliptins carry a low risk of hypoglycaemia
- Although incretins have other effects (eg. GLP-1 reduces glucagon secretion, slows gastric emptying and exerts a satiety effect) the increased levels of incretins achieved with gliptins do not have a major therapeutic impact via such effects

Key features

- Enhance glucose-dependant insulin release
- Require adequate β-cell function
- Low risk of hypoglycaemia (incidence mostly in combination with a sulphonylurea)
- Weight neutral
- Minimal effects on lipid profile

Indications

Type 2 diabetes

- In adults who are inadequately controlled by lifestyle measures and metformin or a sulphonylurea or a TZD
- Can be used in combination with metformin, a sulphonylurea or a TZD (*sitagliptin* is approved for use in triple oral therapy with combinations of these agents)
- Often preferred for patients with erratic meal patterns or other susceptibility to hypoglycaemia eg. religious fasting such as during Ramadan

Table 8.2 Gliptin tablet strengths and doses

Drug	Tablet strength mg	Start dose mg/day	Maximum dose mg/day	Caution
Sitagliptin *Januvia*	100	100	100*	Renal disease
Vildagliptin *Galvus*	50	100 (50 bd)	100#	Hepatic and renal disease

* Consider a lower dose of sulphonylurea when adding sitagliptin
# When adding to a sulphonylurea, vildagliptin 50 mg od is recommended

Dose

- Although gliptins enhance mainly prandial insulin secretion, their low risk of hypoglycaemia means they do not need to be administered with meals

Starting therapy

- Type 2 patients inadequately controlled by lifestyle measures plus one oral agent (metformin, sulphonylurea, TZD)
- Check for contra-indications
- Check liver function (eg. ALT) before starting vildagliptin
- Introduce sitagliptin 100 mg in the morning, or vildagliptin 50 mg twice daily, or vildagliptin 50 mg once daily if adding to sulphonylurea therapy
- Titration is not required in most patients
- Suggest self monitoring of blood glucose occasionally to confirm glycaemic control
- If patient experiences hypoglycaemia:
    - consider reducing one dosage level of the other agent
    - investigate meal and exercise pattern
- If introduction of gliptin produces no benefit:
    - return to previous regimen
    - consider adding an alternative agent
    - consider insulin if hyperglycaemia severe
- If starting or withdrawing any potentially interacting therapy check glycaemic control and adjust regimen if required

Triple therapy

- Sitagliptin can be added in combination with metformin and a sulphonylurea/TZD
- Triple therapy with vildagliptin has not been established

Table 8.3 Efficacy of gliptins	
↓ HbA1c	~0.6 - 1.2% (~6-12 mmol/mol) if starting HbA1c ~8% (~64 mmol/mol)
↓ FPG	0.6-1.2 mmol/L (10-22 mg/dL)
↓ PPG	1-3 mmol/L (18-54 mg/dL)

Contra-indications

- *Moderate or severe renal insufficiency*
- *Significant hepatic disease*
     (eg. serum ALT >3 x ULN for vildagliptin)
- *Cardiac failure*
     (NYHA III-IV) for vildagliptin
- *Pregnancy and breast feeding*
- *Hypersensitivity*
     Hypersensitivity to active ingredient or excipients (check for skin conditions and angioedema)
- *Type 1 diabetes or previous ketosis*

Adverse effects

- *Hypoglycaemia:*
     low risk, rarely severe,
     more likely in combination with a sulphonylurea

Precautions

Table 8.4 Potential drug interactions that could alter glucose-lowering effect of gliptins	
Intrinsic glucose-lowering activity	Other antidiabetic drugs
Intrinsic hyperglycaemic activity	Glucocorticoids and other agents with hyperglycaemic activity
Sitagliptin is eliminated by renal tubular secretion via OAT3. Agents that use or inhibit this transporter (eg. probenecid) could theoretically influence the efficacy of sitagliptin	
Sitagliptin is also a substrate for p-glycoprotein, and inhibitors such as ciclosporin can reduce clearance of sitagliptin, but this does not appear to be a clinically significant effect	
Beta-adrenergic blockers can mask symptoms of hypoglycaemia and reduce counter-regulation	

- Monitor glucose periodically to ensure optimal control maintained
- Ensure patient can recognise and respond to symptoms of hypoglycaemia
- Check periodically for emergence of contra-indications, especially moderate or severe renal insufficiency or significant/severe hepatic disease
- Caution in patients with cardiac failure (vildagliptin not recommended in NYHA III-IV)
- Check skin routinely for any lesions
- Infections (eg. upper respiratory tract) and pancreatic disease have been reported, but no causality established

Discontinue therapy

- If contra-indications develop
- If hypoglycaemia becomes an issue
- If side effects develop or risk of drug interactions

9 THIAZOLIDINEDIONES

Historical developments

Thiazolidinediones (TZDs) are also known as glitazones and PPARγ agonists. TZDs were investigated as glucose-lowering compounds in the early 1980s before PPARγ had been identified. The first TZD, troglitazone (*Romozin*) was introduced and withdrawn in the UK in 1997, due to idiosyncratic hepatotoxicity. This does not appear to be an issue with the two current TZDs, pioglitazone (*Actos*) and rosiglitazone (*Avandia*) which were introduced to the UK in 2000. These agents increase insulin sensitivity for which they are sometimes referred to as 'insulin sensitisers'.

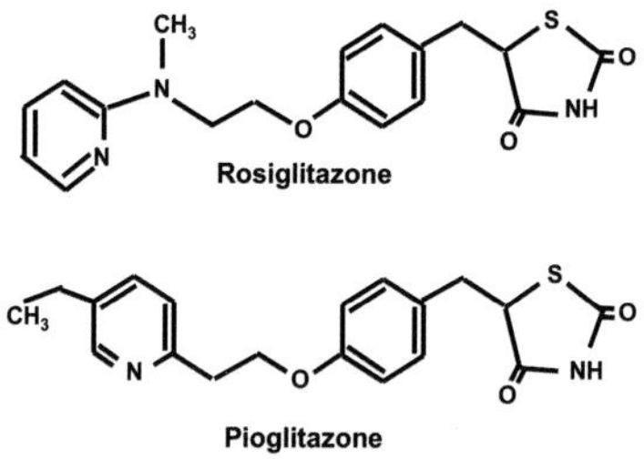

Figure 9.1 Structure of pioglitazone and rosiglitazone

Table 9.1 Pharmacokinetics of TZDs

	Pioglitazone	Rosiglitazone
Absorption	~100% absorbed T_{max} <2 h	~99% absorbed. T_{max} ~1 h
Distribution	>99% protein bound	>99% protein bound
Metabolism	Liver CYP2C8, CYP3A4 Active metabolites	Liver CYP2C8, CYP2C9, Very weakly active metabolites
Elimination	Bile ~55%, t½ 3-7 h (16-24 h)*	Urine ~65%, t½ 3-4 h (100-160 h)*

*(includes metabolites)

Mode of action

* Stimulate the peroxisome proliferator-activated receptor-γ (PPARγ)
* PPARγ is a nuclear receptor that:
    - is strongly expressed in adipose tissue
    - forms a complex with the RXR
    - acts as a transcription factor
    - increases expression of genes affecting adipogenesis, glucose and lipid metabolism, and anti-inflammatory effects
* Stimulation of PPARγ by TZDs:
    - increases formation of small insulin sensitive adipocytes in peripheral adipose depots
    - increases uptake of fatty acids and glucose into these adipocytes
    - decreases circulating fatty acids
    - decreases accumulation of lipids in muscle and liver
    - alters the glucose-fatty acid (Randle) cycle to reduce availability of fatty acids and increase glucose utilisation
* Structural differences between TZDs can affect the selection of genes transcribed and the extent of transcription

Key features

* Increase insulin sensitivity
* Require presence of some insulin for glucose-lowering efficacy
* Slow onset of blood glucose-lowering effect
* Not stimulate insulin secretion
* Not cause overt hypoglycaemia when used as monotherapy
* Variable effects on lipid profile
* Often cause weight gain
* Caution over fluid retention and cardiovascular implications
* Improve several components of 'metabolic syndrome' but contra-indicated in individuals at high risk of cardiac failure

Table 9.2 Gene effects of PPARγ stimulation by TZDs.
The main effect is in adipose tissue, but some of the genes
are activated in other tissues

Adipose tissue	Gene expression
Lipid metabolism	↑ Lipoprotein lipase (LPL) ↑ Fatty acid transporter protein (FATP/CD36) ↑ Adipocyte fatty acid binding protein (aP2) ↑ Acyl-CoA synthetase, ↑ Malic enzyme ↑ Perilipin, ↑ Glycerol kinase ?
Glucose metabolism	↑ GLUT4 (by derepression)
Cortisol production	↓ 11β-HSD1
Adipokines	↓ resistin, ↓ RBP4, ↑adiponectin (↑ leptin ?) ↓ TNFα, ↓ IL-6, ↓CRP, ↓ NFKB ↓ PAI-1, ↓ MMP-9

↑ increase expression; ↓ decrease expression; ? unconfirmed

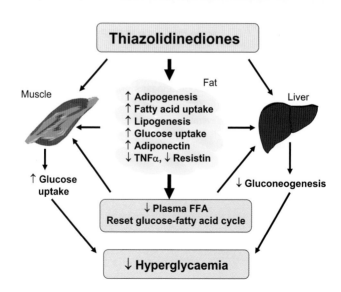

Figure 9.2 Mode of action of TZDs to reduce hyperglycaemia

Table 9.3 Effects of TZDs on the cardiovascular risk indicators of 'metabolic syndrome' *

Effects of TZDs

Insulin resistance	Decrease, mainly via PPARγ agonism
Hyperinsulinaemia	Reduce fasting insulin and proinsulin
Abdominal obesity	Visceral fat little changed Subcutaneous fat usually increased Overall increase body weight
Hyperglycaemia	Improve glycaemic control in type 2 diabetes and IGT
Dyslipidaemia	Variable benefits: both TZDs ↓ FFAs, produce small ↑ HDLc, and decrease the proportion of small (more dense) LDL particles. Pioglitazone can also ↓ TG and ↓ total LDLc
Raised blood pressure	Generally small ↓ BP
Coagulation status	↓ thrombotic risk: ↓ PAI-1, ↓ fibrinogen
Pro-inflammatory markers	↓ some markers e.g. CRP, TNFα, IL-6
Atherosclerosis	↓ some markers eg. adhesion molecules, monocyte attractant protein, metalloproteinases, IM thickness, restenosis and vascular smooth muscle proliferation.

* Note: despite reducing several markers and surrogate measures of CV risk, rosiglitazone has been associated with increased MI in some studies, but this is unsubstantiated in other studies.

↑ increase,   ↓ decrease

Indications

Type 2 diabetes

- In adults who are inadequately controlled by lifestyle measures.
- Often preferred for overweight and obese patients.
- Can be used as monotherapy if metformin contra-indicated or not tolerated.
- Can be used in combination with any other class of oral glucose-lowering agent
- Can be used as triple oral combination with metformin and a sulphonylurea
- *Pioglitazone* can be used with insulin when metformin with insulin is contra-indicated or not tolerated
- *Rosiglitazone* can be used with insulin in exceptional cases and under close supervision.

Dose

- Doses of TZDs reflect their affinity for PPARγ.

Table 9.4 TZD tablet strengths and doses

Drug	Tablet strength mg	Start dose mg/day	Maximum dose mg/day	Caution
Pioglitazone *Actos*	15, 30, 45	15	45	NYHA I-IV
Rosiglitazone *Avandia*	4, 8	4	8	NYHA I-IV

Starting therapy

- Newly diagnosed: trial of lifestyle measures first
- Check for contra-indications
- Check liver function (eg. ALT) before starting
- Introduce once daily in the morning, usually with lowest dose
- Due to slow onset of glucose-lowering activity, full effect of any dose may take 4-8 weeks: thus up-titrate by increasing dose at 4-8 week intervals, initially based on FPG

- Self-monitoring of blood glucose can be helpful
- If patient shows no benefit or poor response (eg. ↓ HbA1c <0.5% by 6 months) NICE suggests discontinue and switch to an alternative therapy.
- If patient shows rapid weight gain or signs of possible fluid retention, return to previous dose (discontinue if not resolve)
- If patient experiences hypoglycaemia (very uncommon as monotherapy), reduce one dosage level
- If starting or withdrawing any potentially interacting therapy check glycaemic control: due to slow reversal of effect consider altering the interacting drug if this is for temporary use

Combination therapy

- TZDs can be added when monotherapy with another agent does not achieve or sustain adequate glycaemic control
- Other types of antidiabetic agents can be added when TZD monotherapy is inadequate
- TZDs can be used part of a triple therapy regimen
- TZDs can be used with insulin but require extra caution: likely reduction of insulin dose and increased risk of fluid retention. Insulin + rosiglitazone - only in exceptional cases, with close supervision

Table 9.5 Efficacy of TZDs	
↓ HbA1c	~0.6-2% (~6-22 mmol/mol) if starting HbA1c ~8% (~64 mmol/mol).
↓ FPG	2-3 mmol/L (36-54 mg/dL)
Lipids	↓ FFA; pioglitazone also ↓ TG
Other	Basal insulin concentrations unchanged or slightly reduced Overt hypoglycaemia unlikely as monotherapy

Contra-indications

- **Cardiac failure**

   Any evidence of cardiac failure (NYHA I-IV see chapter 15). Avoid *rosiglitazone* in ACS

- **Significant hepatic disease**

   Eg. serum ALT >2.5 x ULN or known liver disease. Note that under carefully monitored conditions TZDs have been reported to improve NAFLD (NASH).

- **Pregnancy and breast feeding**

   Not recommended

- **Hypersensitivity**

   Known previous hypersensitivity to TZDs or excipients.

- **Type 1 diabetes or previous ketosis.**

Adverse effects

- **Body weight gain**

   Typically ↑1-4kg, usually stabilising after ~6-12 months

- **Fluid retention**

   Increased risk of fluid retention and dilutional anaemia

- **Congestive heart disease**

   Increased risk of congestive heart disease

- **Hypoglycaemia**

   Combination therapy may be associated with hypoglycaemia

- **Fractures**

   Risk of bone fractures, mainly in older women

Precautions

- Check for evidence of oedema, congestive heart disease, or development of any cardiac contra-indications
- Periodic (eg. annual) check of liver function: stop if ALT >3 x ULN
- Caution in patients with severe renal insufficiency
- Monitor glucose periodically after titration to ensure optimal control maintained

- Risk of hypoglycaemia in combination with other antidiabetic agents
- Caution over use of high doses in older women with known low bone density
- Caution if used with insulin (increased risk of oedema, monitor cardiac status): insulin with *rosiglitazone* only in exceptional cases
- Altered visual acuity: check for signs of macular oedema
- Ovulation can resume in individuals with PCOS

Table 9.6 Potential drug interactions that can alter the glucose-lowering effect of TZDs

Intrinsic glucose-lowering activity	Other antidiabetic drugs
Intrinsic hyperglycaemic effect	Glucocorticoids
Increased hepatic metabolism (decreased glucose-lowering effect)	Rifampicin (inducer of CYP2C8)
Decreased hepatic metabolism (increased glucose-lowering effect)	Gemfibrozil (inhibitor of CYP2C8)

Beta-adrenergic blockers can mask symptoms of hypoglycaemia and reduce counter-regulation

Discontinue therapy

- If contra-indications develop
    - particularly cardiac symptoms (*rosiglitazone* is contra-indicated in ACS)
    - deteriorating liver function, ALT >3 x ULN
- If decrease in HbA1c <0.5% in 6 months (NICE guideline 87)
- If rapid initial weight gain associated with fluid retention
- If side effects develop or evidence of drug interactions

10 ACARBOSE

Historical developments

Acarbose (*Glucobay*) is the only alpha-glucosidase inhibitor (AGI) used in the UK. Taken with food, it binds to intestinal alpha-glucosidase enzymes and slows carbohydrate digestion. Acarbose was identified as a metabolite in cultures of actinomycete fungi and introduced in the UK in 1993.

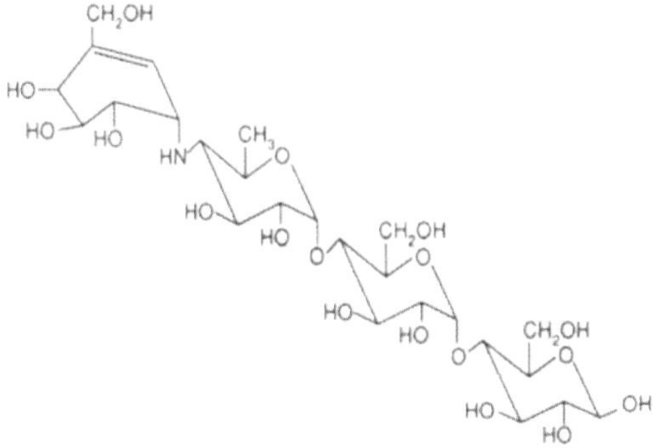

Figure 10.1 Structure of acarbose

Table 10.1 Pharmacokinetics of acarbose	
Absorption	Acts within intestine 1-2% absorbed as intact drug ~30% absorbed as intestinal metabolites
Metabolism	~50% metabolised in intestine by amylases and bacteria
Elimination	Unabsorbed drug and metabolites eliminated faeces Absorbed drug and metabolites eliminated in urine in 24 h without systemic effects

Mode of action

- Slows the digestion of complex carbohydrate and sucrose in the small intestine:
  - this slows the rate of absorption of glucose and defers the process further along the intestine
  - by extending the postprandial period, the height of the hyperglycaemic excursion is reduced.
- Acarbose acts by high affinity binding to alpha-glucosidase enzymes in the brush border membranes of enterocytes:
  - it competitively prevents binding and cleavage of disaccharides and oligosaccaharides into monosaccharides
- The blood glucose-lowering efficacy of acarbose is mainly due to reduced postprandial hyperglycaemia
- The reduced hyperglycaemia is often associated with a reduced prandial insulin response
- Note - for acarbose to be effective meals must contain a substantial amount of complex carbohydrate (acarbose is ineffective against dietary monosaccharides).

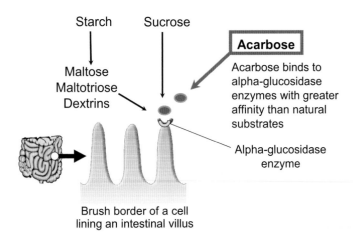

Figure 10.2 Mode of action of acarbose
Acarbose competes with intestinal alpha-glucosidase enzymes, slowing carbohydrate digestion

Key features

- Slows intestinal carbohydrate digestion and thereby slows rate of availability for absorption
- Acts mainly to reduce postprandial glucose excursion
- Not stimulate insulin secretion
- Not cause hypoglycaemia
- Weight neutral
- May improve postprandial lipid profile

Indications

Type 2 diabetes

- In adults who are inadequately controlled by lifestyle measures alone or with other oral antidiabetic agents
- More often preferred for patients with erratic meal patterns or other susceptibility to hypoglycaemia
- More useful against postprandial (rather than basal) hyperglycaemia
- Can be used in combination with other classes of glucose-lowering agents

Dose

- Dose 50 mg, 100 mg tablets od, bd or tds
- Maximum permitted daily dose 200 mg tds
- Acarbose should always be taken with meals rich in complex carbohydrate

Starting therapy

- Newly diagnosed: trial of lifestyle measures first
- Check for contra-indications (especially gastrointestinal)
- Take acarbose tablets immediately before a main meal, chewed or swallowed whole
- Start with 50 mg at one meal
- Titrate up to 50 mg with two then three meals over 1-2 months
- Monitor postprandial glycaemia and further titrate to 100 mg tds if required and tolerated

- If required and tolerated consider further titration to 200 mg tds.
- Suggest intermittent self-monitoring of blood glucose if possible to check efficacy (usually 1-2 h after beginning the meal)
- If patient experiences gastrointestinal side effects:
    - reduce or omit dosage at one or more meals
- If dose titration produces no benefit:
    - return to previous dosage
    - consider adding agent with different cellular mode of action
- If starting or withdrawing any potentially interacting therapy check glycaemic control and adjust regimen as required

Combination therapy

- Acarbose can be added when monotherapy or combination therapy with other antidiabetic agents does not achieve or sustain adequate glycaemic control
- Although acarbose is not specifically indicated for use with insulin, it has been used in insulin-treated patients (see SPC and BNF) to reduce postprandial hyperglycaemia, and to prolong digestion in order to reduce risk of interprandial hypoglycaemia

Table 10.2 Efficacy of acarbose	
↓ HbA1c	~0.5% (~6 mmol/mol), occasionally >1% (>11 mmol/mol)
↓ FPG	~0.5 mmol/L (~9 mg/dL)
↓ PPG	1-4 mmol/L (18-72 mg/dL)

Contra-indications

- *GI disorders*
  Especially inflammatory bowel disease, colonic ulceration, obstructive diseases or predisposition to obstruction, or states that could be aggravated by increased gas formation
- *Significant liver disease*
- *Severe renal impairment*
  Creatinine clearance <25 mL/min/1.73m^2
- *Pregnancy and breast feeding*
- *Hypersensitivity*
  Known hypersensitivity to acarbose or excipients
- *Type 1 diabetes or previous ketosis*

Adverse effects

- *Hypoglycaemia*
  Rare when used as monotherapy
  More likely in combination with other antidiabetic drugs
- *GI intolerance*
  GI intolerance or aggravation of GI disease
- *Abnormal liver function*
  This is very rare

Drug interactions

- Drugs affecting GI motility could potentially alter the effectiveness and GI side effects of acarbose
- Intestinal adsorbents (eg. charcoal) and digestive enzyme preparations (eg. amylase, pancreatin) could reduce efficacy of acarbose
- Colestyramine can enhance the effects of acarbose

Precautions

- Monitor glucose periodically during and after titration to check glycaemic control
- Ensure patient can recognise and respond to symptoms of hypoglycaemia
- Caution, check for emergence of contra-indications, notably gastrointestinal, renal and hepatic disease

Discontinue therapy

- If contra-indications develop
- If substantial side effects or risk of drug interactions occur

11 FIXED-DOSE COMBINATIONS

Historical developments

Combinations of differently acting antidiabetic agents are frequently required to address the progressive deterioration of glycaemic control in type 2 diabetes. Fixed-dose combination (FDC) tablets are 'single' tablets that contain the active ingredients of commonly used antidiabetic combinations. FDCs are gaining increasing acceptance.

Table 11.1 Fixed-dose 'single' tablet combinations of antidiabetic drugs in the UK

Tablet™	Components	Strengths (mg)
Avandamet	metformin + rosiglitazone	500:2; 1000:2; 1000:4
Competact	metformin + pioglitazone	850:15
Eucreas	metformin + vildagliptin	850:50; 1000:50

Properties

- FDCs are formulated to have similar bioequivalence properties to the two agents as separate tablets
- Thus FDCs have pharmacokinetic and pharmacodynamic properties that are not generally distinguishable from the two agents given as separate tablets.
- The range of dosage strengths available as FDCs includes most of the commonly used dosage strengths as single tablets

Uses of FDCs

- Convenience, especially to reduce the pill burden in type 2 diabetes
- Can improve adherance in some individuals with a high pill burden: this in turn improves their glycaemic control
- May facilitate use of two drugs at lower doses than one drug

at a high dose: this approach can be used to reduce the side effects associated with a high dose of one drug
- It is often advised that agents are introduced 'individually' to assist dose titration and to help identify the source of side effects. However, many type 2 diabetes patients will already be taking the proposed combination, and the side effects of most common antidiabetic agents are distinctive and well recognised

Indications, efficacy and contra-indications

- Indications, efficacy and contra-indications for an FDC are the same as for the two active ingredients as separate tablets (Note that contra-indications must be respected for each active ingredient)
- Some FDCs can be used as part of a triple therapy regimen as indicated for the separate tablets
- Tolerability, adverse events and drug interactions are the same as for each of the two active ingredients, but may be less limiting if lower doses of the combination are used

Switching to FDC therapy

- Patients already taking a particular antidiabetic combination as separate tablets can be switched to the same doses of each agent as FDCs, usually without alteration of the administration schedule
- If the exact dose equivalent is not available as FDC, select the nearest lower dose and titrate up if necessary

Starting FDC therapy

- This will usually involve metformin-treated patients for whom a second agent is to be added
- Select the current dose schedule for metformin with the lowest available dose of the second agent
- Follow the same procedure as if adding a separate tablet, ie. monitor glucose control and titrate up to a higher strength if required

- If initiating FDC therapy as first pharmacological therapy follow the same approach as starting metformin, respecting contra-indications for both agents in the combination
- Appreciate that combination of metformin with a TZD may take longer to exert its glucose-lowering effect than metformin alone, and extend the titration time as appropriate to the TZD

Discontinue FDC therapy

- If contra-indications to either active component develop
- If an increase in dose produces no benefit or side effects become limiting revert to the previous dose
- Consider either additional (triple) therapy or use of a different therapy which may need to be insulin

12 GLP-1 AGONISTS

Historical developments

The incretin hormone GLP-1 exerts a glucose-dependent insulinotropic effect. However it is very rapidly degraded in the circulation (t½ 1-2 min) by DPP4, which precludes its use as a subcutaneously injected therapy.

GLP-1 agonists comprise two peptides based on GLP-1 that have a modified structure to confer resistance to breakdown by DPP4. These agonists act by stimulating the GLP-1 receptor and producing a similar profile of effects to GLP-1. They are administered by sc injection: exenatide (*Byetta*) introduced 2007 is given twice daily and liraglutide (*Victoza*) introduced 2009 is given once daily.

Structure
* Exenatide has ~53% homology with native GLP-1 and is modified at the N-terminus to prevent degradation by DPP4
* Liraglutide has ~97% homology with native GLP-1. It has a palmitoyl fatty acid chain added to enable self-association and attachment to albumin in the circulation, which protects against degradation by DPP4

DPP4*

⇓

Human GLP-1	HA EGT FTS DV SSYLE GQAAK EFIAW LVKGR (7-36) amide
Human GLP-1	HA EGT FTS DV SSYLE GQAAK EFIAW LVKGR G (7-37)
Exenatide	HG EGT FTS DL SKQME EEAVR LFIEW LKNGG PSSGA PPPSG
Liraglutide	HA EGT FTS DV SSYLE GQAAK EFIAW LVRGR G

E--palmitoyl----albumin

* Peptides with an alanine (A) residue at position N-2 are cleaved by dipeptidyl peptidase 4 (DPP4).

Figure 12.1 Structure of GLP-1, exenatide and liraglutide

Table 12.1 Pharmacokinetics of GLP-1 agonists		
	Exenatide	**Liraglutide**
Absorption	sc injection T_{max} ~2 h	sc injection T_{max} 8-12 h
Distribution	Not plasma protein bound	>98% protein bound
Metabolism	Mostly removed by glomerular filtration with subsequent proteolysis	<14% circulating metabolites (due to metabolism in circulation)
Elimination	Mostly urine $t\frac{1}{2}$ ~2.4 h	Breakdown products in urine and faeces $t\frac{1}{2}$ ~13 h

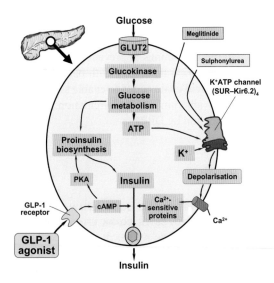

Figure 12.2   Mode of action of GLP-1 agonists to potentiate insulin release by pancreatic β-cells

Mode of action

- GLP-1 agonists exert similar effects to native GLP-1, but the effects are more pronounced due to the extended half-lives of the agonists
- The main glucose-lowering effect is to enhance glucose-mediated insulin secretion
  - GLP-1 acts via a specific G-protein coupled receptor on the pancreatic β-cell to potentiate the secretion of insulin
- The insulinotropic effect of GLP-1 requires that insulin secretion has already been initiated by raised circulating nutrients (mainly glucose) after a meal, ie. enhance prandial insulin secretion
  - GLP-1 will also potentiate insulin secretion initiated by pharmacological agents such as sulphonylureas
- Other effects of GLP-1 that contribute to its glucose-lowering effect are:
  - decreased secretion of glucagon by pancreatic α-cells; this is a glucose dependent effect, so it does not prevent the counter-regulatory response to hypoglycaemia
  - reduced rate of gastric emptying, centrally mediated, which slows the rate of digestion and assists glucose-lowering (but can cause nausea)
  - satiety effect, centrally mediated which appears to contribute to long-term weight loss
- Note, whereas sulphonylureas and meglitinides can initiate insulin secretion at low glucose concentrations, GLP-1 agonists potentiate insulin secretion that has been initiated by raised nutrient concentrations or other drugs
- Thus GLP-1 agonists carry a low risk of hypoglycaemia
- GLP-1 receptors have been identified in the vasculature and may assist a small decrease in blood pressure

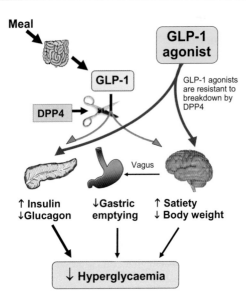

Figure 12.3 Mode of action of GLP-1 and GLP-1 agonists.
GLP-1 and its agonists mainly reduce prandial hyperglycaemia by
potentiating glucose-induced insulin secretion, reducing glucagon
secretion, slowing gastric emptying and exerting a satiety effect.

Key features

- Enhance glucose-dependent insulin release
- Insulinotropic effect requires adequate β-cell function
- Low risk of hypoglycaemia (mostly with sulphonylurea)
- Weight-lowering effect
- Minimal effects on lipid profile

Indications

Type 2 diabetes

- In adults who are inadequately controlled by lifestyle measures, metformin and/or a sulphonylurea
- Can be used in combination with metformin and/or a sulphonylurea
- Liraglutide can also be used in combination with metformin plus TZD: SPC states limited experience of exenatide with a TZD
- Often preferred for obese patients and those considered at particular risk of hypoglycaemia (NICE suggests use mainly in patients with BMI >35 kg/m^2)

Dose

- *Exenatide* dose is 5 μg or 10 μg twice daily by sc injection
  Solution contains 0.25 mg/mL (5 μg dose = 20 μL ; 10μg dose = 40 μL) in non-adjustable preloaded pen
- *Liraglutide* doses are 0.6, 1.2 mg or 1.8 mg once daily by sc injection
  Solution contains 6 mg/mL (0.6 mg dose = 100 μL, 1.2 mg dose = 200 μL, 1.8 mg dose = 300 μL) in adjustable preloaded pen
- Choice of injection sites same as for insulin (abdomen, thigh, upper arm)

Table 12.2 GLP-1 agonists: strengths and doses for sc injection.

Drug	Injection solution	Start dose	Maximum daily dose	Injection time
Exenatide *Byetta*	0.25 mg/mL	5 μg bd	10 μg bd	Up to 1 h before two main meals*
Liraglutide *Victoza*	6 mg/mL	0.6 mg od	1.8 mg od	Once daily at any time**

*Usually breakfast and evening meals, but can be any two meals taken >6 h apart
** Preferable to use the same time of day each day

Starting therapy

- Type 2 patients inadequately controlled by lifestyle measures plus one or two oral agents (metformin, sulphonylurea, TZD)
- Check for contra-indications (principally renal status)
- *Exenatide* start 5 μg injection twice daily (pre-breakfast and pre-evening meal) for 1 month
  - if control inadequate and drug tolerated (initial nausea) increase dose to 10 μg dose twice daily
- *Liraglutide* start 0.6 mg injection once daily (usually morning) for 1-4 wks
  - if control inadequate and drug tolerated (initial nausea) increase dose to 1.2 mg once daily
  - titrate further to 1.8 mg once daily if required
- Self monitoring of blood glucose may be helpful during drug titration, especially with a sulphonylurea, and periodically thereafter to ensure control maintained
- Ensure patients can recognise and respond to symptoms of hypoglycaemia, and appreciate potential GI side effects and reports of pancreatitis
- If patient experiences hypoglycaemia:
  - reduce one dosage level of the other agent
  - or reduce dose level of GLP-1 agonist
  - and investigate meal and exercise pattern
- If introduction of GLP-1 agonist produces no benefit:
  - return to previous regimen
  - consider adding alternative agent
  - consider insulin if hyperglycaemia is severe
- If starting or withdrawing any potentially interacting therapy check glycaemic control and adjust regimen if required

Triple therapy

- Exenatide and liraglutide can be used with metformin and sulphonylurea
- Liraglutide can also be used with metformin and a TZD

Table 12.3 Efficacy of GLP-1 agonists	
↓ HbA1c	~0.6 - 1.5% (~6-16 mmol/mol) if starting HbA1c ~8.5% (~70 mmol/mol)
↓ FPG	0.7-2.5 mmol/L (13-45 mg/dL)
↓ PPG	1.5-3 mmol/L (27-54 mg/dL)
↓ Body weight	1-4 kg over 6-12 months
Hypoglyceamia	Low risk - more likely when given in combination with a sulphonylurea

A 6-month study comparing liraglutide (1.8 mg od) with exenatide (10 μg bd) reported a slightly greater reduction in HbA1c with liraglutide (↓ 1.12 %; - 12 mmol/mol) than exenatide (↓ 0.79 %; - 9 mmol/mol).

Contra-indications

- *Renal impairment*

  Exenatide is not recommended in severe renal impairment (creatinine clearance <30 mL/min)

  Liraglutide is not recommended in moderate renal impairment (creatinine clearance <60 mL/min)

- *Significant GI disease*

  Especially gastroparesis (and inflammatory bowel disease with liraglutide)

- *Pregnancy and breast feeding*

- *Hypersensitivity*

  Hypersensitivity to active ingredient or excipients (check for skin conditions)

- *Type 1 diabetes or previous ketosis*

  Patients requiring insulin due to β-cell failure

Adverse effects

- *Hypoglycaemia*

  Risk is low, very rarely severe, more likely in combination with a sulphonylurea

- *Nausea*
    Is dose-dependent and usually transient:.
    at least one episode experienced by 20-40% of patients
    during initial 2 months of therapy
- *Injection site reactions*
    These have been reported in 2-5% of patients
- *Pancreatitis, angiodema, thyroid issues*
    Acute pancreatitis and angioedema have been reported
    rarely during long-term use, but it is not clear if these are
    drug-related
    Liraglutide has been associated with an increased
    occurrence of raised calcitonin and adverse thyroid events
    (~0.5-1% of patients)

Drug interactions

- Reschedule administration times of any concurrent
    medications affected by delayed gastric emptying, eg.
    - drugs requiring threshold concentrations for efficacy
        such as antibiotics,
    - drugs degraded in the stomach
- If taking warfarin suggest initial extra monitoring of INR
- If taking a statin suggest check lipid profile
- GLP-1 agonists do not appear to exert clinically meaningful
    effects on oral glucose-lowering drugs
- Beta-adrenergic blockers can mask symptoms of
    hypoglycaemia and reduce counter-regulation

Precautions

- Monitor glucose periodically to ensure optimal control
    maintained
- Ensure patient can recognise and respond to symptoms of
    hypoglycaemia
- Observe for symptoms of emergent gastrointestinal disease or
    pancreatitis
- Check periodically for emergence of contra-indications,
    especially renal insufficiency

- Caution with liraglutide in hepatic disease and congestive heart failure: check thyroid
- Antibodies to GLP-1 agonists have been detected:
    - in up to 38% of patients receiving exenatide
    - in 5-15% receiving liraglutide.
- Antibody titres may recede during long-term use and efficacy is not usually significantly affected, but may lead to reduced efficacy and drug withdrawal in a very small proportion of chronically treated patients.

Discontinue therapy

- If contra-indications develop
- If hypoglycaemia becomes an issue
- If GI symptoms persist or GI disease develops or symptoms of pancreatitis emerge
- If side effects persist or there is significant risk of drug interactions

13 INSULINS

Historical developments

After the introduction of insulin therapy (1922) pork and beef insulins were used until the introduction of human insulin (1981) and insulin analogues (1996). Insulin therapy is essential to maintain life in type 1 diabetes (absolute lack of endogenous insulin), and it is often required to control the hyperglycaemia in advanced states of type 2 diabetes.

Structure

Natural human insulin is:
- a 51 amino acid peptide
- comprising two chains (A-chain 21 amino acids and B- chain 30 amino acids) linked by disulphide bridges
- synthesised by the pancreatic β-cells as a single chain peptide (proinsulin) which is broken and folded into the A- and B-chains of insulin with separation of C-peptide

Table 13.1 Types of insulin

Type	Produced by
Animal	Extraction from porcine and bovine pancreas
Human semi-synthetic	Chemically (enzymatically) modified pork (*emp*)
Human biosynthetic*	Recombinant DNA in yeast or bacteria
Analogue*	Recombinant DNA in yeast or bacteria

*Synthesis is via proinsulin or separate chains that are joined chemically:
- pyr = proinsulin yeast recombinant
- prb = proinsulin recombinant bacteria
- crb = chain recombinant bacteria

Natural insulins

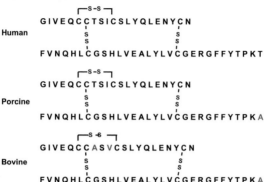

Rapid-acting analogue insulins

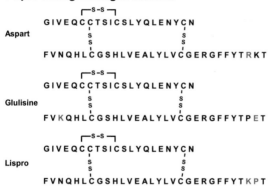

Long-acting analogue insulins

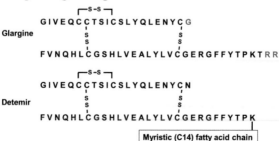

Myristic (C14) fatty acid chain

Figure 13.1 Amino acid sequences of animal, human and analogue insulins

Table 13.2 Summary of amino acid substitutions in animal and analogue insulins compared with human insulin

Type of insulin	Amino acid substitution
Animal	
Bovine	A8-Ala, A10 Val, B30-Ala
Porcine	B30-Ala
Analogue	
Aspart (*NovoRapid*)	B28-Asp
Glulisine (*Apidra*)	B3-Lys, B29-Glu
Lispro (*Humalog*)	B28-Lys, B29-Pro
Detemir (*Levemir*)	B29-Lys with attached fatty acid chain (myristic acid), B30-Thr deleted
Glargine (*Lantus*)	A21-Gly, B31-Arg, B32-Arg

Table 13.3 Pharmacokinetics of insulins

Natural (endogenous) human insulin is:

secreted by the pancreas into the portal circulation

rapidly degraded in the circulation (plasma t½ ~2-5 min)

mainly removed from the circulation by the liver and kidney, and eliminated in the bile and urine

Therapeutic insulin preparations:

have different rates of onset and duration of action

have different formulations and/or different structures which alter the rates at which they are absorbed from the subcutaneous injection site and become freely available in the circulation

once free in the circulation are quickly degraded and removed in the same ways as natural insulin

Strength and potency

- All insulin preparations are supplied at a strength of
  U-100 = 100 Units/mL
  This means 100 Units/mL of glucose-lowering activity
- 1 unit of activity is equivalent to 37.5 µg (6 nmol) of pure natural human insulin
- Thus U-100 human insulin contains 3.75 mg/mL (0.6 mmol/L)
- This equates to a potency for human insulin of 26 Units/mg
- Insulin analogues have different affinities for insulin receptors and some other receptors (eg. IGF-1 receptors), but these analogues are formulated to deliver 100 Units/mL of glucose-lowering activity (eg. glargine 3.64 mg/mL; detemir   14.2 mg/mL)
- Under special circumstances high strength (U-500) insulin formulations can be requested
- In Europe biphasic insulins are defined by the % rapid/short component first (eg, 30/70 is 30% rapid/short and 70% intermediate/long): the opposite nomenclature is used in some countries (eg. USA)

Classification

Insulins are usually classified according to
- Onset and duration of action
  - rapid , short, intermediate, long
- Way in which they are used
  - basal, bolus (prandial), biphasic (pre-mixed)

Table 13.4 Classification of insulins by time of onset, peak and duration of action

	Action		
	Onset	Peak (h)	Duration (h)
Rapid	10 min	1-3	3-4
Short	½-1 h	2-5	6-8
Intermediate	1-4 h	3-12	10-22
Long	2-8 h	4-20	18-24+

Table 13.5 Classification of insulins according to use

	Other names	Use as sc injection	Types of insulin
Basal	Background Maintenance	Once or twice daily, Morning and/or evening	Intermediate Long-acting
Bolus	Prandial Meal-time	Before or with main meals	Rapid-acting Short-acting
Biphasic	Pre-mixed Mixtures	Usually twice daily Morning and evening	Mix of rapid/short with intermediate/long

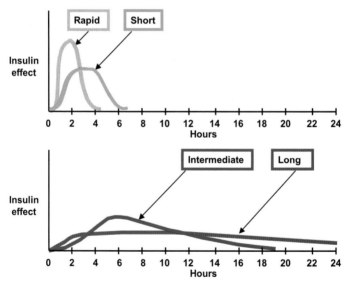

Figure 13.2   Time course profiles for glucose-lowering
effects of insulins

Formulation and duration of action

The speed of onset and duration of action of insulin preparations has been modified using protamine, zinc, mixtures and analogues.

Protamine

This is a fish sperm protein which binds with insulin in a non-covalent manner to reduce the solubility of insulin in the subcutaneous depot after injection. This delays absorption and prolongs the duration of action.

Isophane (NPH) insulin contains insulin and protamine in a stoichiometric proportion (ie. all insulin is bound, none is free).

Zinc

The presence of excess zinc in acetate buffer facilitates the crystallisation of insulin to form a suspension: crystallisation slows the dissolution of insulin from the subcutaneous depot after injection. The rate of dissolution varies according to the size, shape and aggregation of the crystals.

Lente insulin such as Hypurin Bovine Lente is a suspension of insulin-zinc crystals.

Mixtures

Pre-mixed insulins contain protamine-insulin with no excess zinc (intermediate-acting), and an excess of free insulin (not crystallised; short- or rapid-acting) which then remains separate.

Mixtard 30 contains 30% short-acting insulin and 70% isophane. Insuman Comb 50 contains 50% soluble insulin and 50% isophane.

Rapid-acting analogues

Regular (neutral, soluble) human insulin self-associates into hexamers with zinc. These dissociate in the subcutaneous depot into dimers and then monomers which enter the circulation. Minor changes to the amino acid sequence of the insulin molecule can prevent or reduce association into hexamers so that dissociation to monomers is rapid, enabling fast entry into the circulation.

Insulin Lispro is a rapid-acting analogue with a reduced capacity to form dimers.

Long-acting analogues

Minor changes to the amino acid sequence can change the pH at which insulin self-associates, such that stronger self-association in the subcutaneous depots will slow the rate of dissociation and entry into the circulation.

Insulin Glargine is a long-acting analogue with minimal self-association in acid solution in the vial, but forms microprecipitates in the slightly alkaline subcutaneous depot. The microprecipitates dissociate slowly to produce a prolonged steady entry into the circulation.

Insulin Detemir is a long-acting analogue with a fatty acid (myristic acid) attached: this promotes self-association in the subcutaneous depot and binds to albumin in the circulation, slowing entry into the circulation and prolonging the plasma half-life.

Mode of action

- Insulin acts by binding to receptors found in the plasma membranes of most cells
- Binding triggers a diversity of intra-cellular signalling pathways
- These pathways control gene expression and also directly alter the activity of enzymes and transporters involved in nutrient metabolism
- Insulin exerts general anabolic effects and has an important role in cell division and differentiation

The main metabolic effects of insulin lower blood glucose by:
- ↓ hepatic glucose output
- ↑ peripheral glucose uptake, storage and metabolism
- ↓ lipolysis

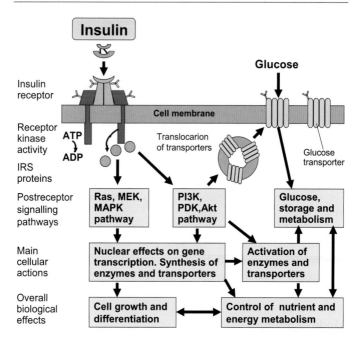

Figure 13.3   The cellular mode of action of insulin

Table 13.6 The main effects of insulin on nutrient metabolism

Effect	Main tissues
↑ Glucose uptake	Muscle, fat
↑ Glycogen synthesis	Muscle, liver
↑ Glycolysis	Muscle, liver, fat
↓ Gluconeogenesis	Liver
↓ Lipolysis	Liver, fat
↑ Lipogenesis	Fat
↑ Amino acid uptake	Muscle
↑ Protein synthesis	Muscle, liver
↓ Protein catabolism	Muscle

Key features

- Subcutaneous injections, once or several times daily
- Requires compatibility with lifestyle routine
- Self-monitoring of blood glucose advised
- High risk of hypoglycaemia
- Weight gain common
- Minor benefits to lipid profile

Indications

Type 1 diabetes
- *Type 1* diabetes at diagnosis

Type 2 diabetes
- *Type 2* diabetes inadequately controlled by lifestyle measures and other antidiabetic medications, or if particularly symptomatic (eg. severely hyperglycaemic, osmotic symptoms, marked unintentional weight loss)
- *Type 2* diabetes patients who require insulin due to co-morbidities (eg. renal or hepatic disease, severe neuropathy), contra-indications or intolerance to other medications, inter-current illness, investigations or surgery, before and during pregnancy and lactation (all with appropriate caution)
- Can be used in combination with metformin, a sulphonylurea and/or other antidiabetic medication where approved as double or triple therapy

Dose and regimen

- Insulin dose is highly dependent on pathophysiological status, type of insulin and regimen selected, preference and circumstances of patient.
- The main subcutaneous insulin injection regimens are:
  - basal
  - basal-bolus
  - biphasic
- Other subcutaneous regimens are occasionally used eg. pre-prandial insulin only in type 2 patients, usually for support during acute illness

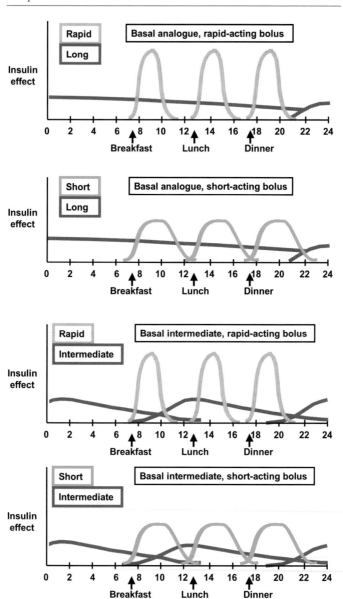

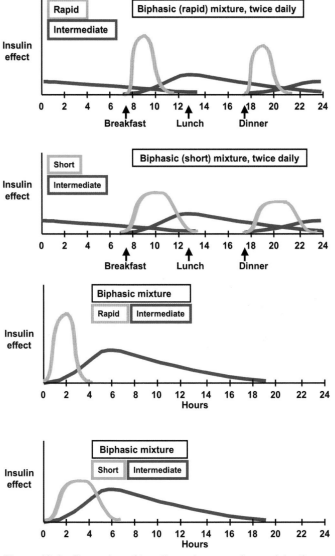

Figure 13.4   Examples of insulin regimens using sc injections of insulins with different rates of onset and durations of action

107

- iv infusion or sc injection, and sometimes intra-muscular injection are given in the treatment of ketoacidosis and hyperosmotic non-ketotic emergencies
- Continuous subcutaneous insulin infusion (CSII) in patients (usually type 1) experiencing significant difficulties with standard regimens and needing an insulin profile that more rigorously mimics the normal endogenous profile

Table 13.7 Subcutaneous insulin regimens

	Injection times	Suited for
Basal	Usually once daily in the morning Sometimes twice daily May include use of oral antidiabetic agents in type 2 patients	Mostly type 2 patients inadequately controlled on other agents Once daily often used to initiate insulin and for short-term cover during inter-current illness
Basal-bolus	Multiple daily injections of insulin (MDI), *viz*: basal insulin (intermediate/long) usually once daily in the morning or evening, and a bolus (rapid/short) before each of the main meals	Preferred for type 1 patients Less frequently used in type 2 patients
Biphasic	Mixtures (usually 'pre-mixed') of rapid/short with intermediate/long usually taken before breakfast and before the evening meal	Suitable for type 1 and 2 patients

Combination of insulin with oral agents

Type 2 diabetes

One or more oral antidiabetic agents may be continued when insulin is introduced in type 2 diabetes. Increased risk of hypoglycaemia requires that the choice and timing of administration of these agents is appropriately harmonised with daily routine

- Insulin with metformin
  - has been used to improve glycaemic control and reduce insulin requirement by improving insulin action. Metformin can reduce insulin-associated weight gain
- Insulin with a TZD
  - can be used if metformin is inappropriate: this combination can substantially reduce insulin requirement but may increase weight gain and enhance risk of oedema. ***Check for any deterioration in cardiac status.*** Insulin should only be added to established rosiglitazone therapy in exceptional circumstances under close supervision
- Insulin with a sulphonylurea
  - has been used to improve glycaemic control when there is sufficient remaining β-cell function: the sulphonylurea increases insulin secretion which boosts the delivery of insulin to the liver to reduce hepatic glucose output
- Insulin with acarbose
  - can be used to prolong meal digestion and smooth the day glucose profile: acarbose may be helpful in insulin-treated patients to reduce interprandial hypoglycaemia.

Starting insulin injections

- This always requires substantial psychological and educational support
- Select a regimen in full consultation with the patient and adapt as appropriate to patient circumstances
- Emphasise importance of lifestyle measures
- Ensure patient is able to recognise and respond to symptoms of hypoglycaemia
- May need to deal with special issues of anxiety or needle phobia
- After initial intervention with insulin, glycaemic control may be very substantially improved for several weeks or months ('honeymoon period') in type 1 patients: this defers the full dose titration process

Children and adolescents - type 1 diabetes
- Should only be undertaken by specialists
- Usually requires prior or concurrent management of acute presentation
- Suggest start basal insulin at 0.1 Units/kg once daily
- The honeymoon period may slow or delay dose titration
- Up-titrate cautiously, usually 1 Unit/day every 1-2 days, based on daily glucose monitoring
- Introduce bolus insulin at 1 Unit/meal as/when appropriate or switch to biphasic (pre-mixed) twice daily with about two thirds of the daily dose in the morning and one third in the evening
- Provide necessary education and support for patient and family

Adults – type 1 diabetes
- Address acute conditions and co-existent morbidities
- For young adults with suspected or confirmed type 1 diabetes, suggest start basal insulin at 6-10 Units/day (for older and heavier patients consider the upper end of the range)
- The honeymoon period may slow or delay dose titration
- Up-titrate carefully, usually 1-2 Units/day based on daily glucose monitoring
- As/when appropriate, introduce bolus insulin at 1-2 Units/meal: aim to give about ½ total daily dose as basal and ½ as bolus doses divided between three meals
- Alternatively switch to biphasic (pre-mixed) twice daily: usually aim for about two thirds of the daily dose in the morning and one third before/with the evening meal
- Typical total daily dose for a type 1 adult is 20-50 Units, being towards the upper end if overweight and the lower end with renal or hepatic disease

Adults – type 2 diabetes
- Address acute conditions and co-existent morbidities
- Continue metformin if already prescribed: consider carefully the potential value of continuing any other antidiabetic therapies

- If HbA1c > 8% (64 mmol/mol) suggest start basal insulin at 10-12 Units/day
- If HbA1c < 8% (64 mmol/mol) suggest start basal insulin at 6 Units/day
- Up-titrate 2-4 Units/day based on daily glucose monitoring: obese patients can usually be increased at 4 Units/day
- If inappropriate prandial hyperglycaemic excursions consider introducing bolus insulin at 2 Units/meal or consider adding low-dose insulin-releasing agent
- Alternatively consider switching to biphasic (pre-mixed) twice daily with slightly >½ the daily dose before/with breakfast and <½ before/with the evening meal
- Typical total daily dose for a type 2 adult is 20-80 Units, being towards the upper end if obese and the lower end with renal or hepatic disease

Continuous Subcutaneous Insulin Infusion (CSII)

- Patients to be considered for CSII should be referred to a specialist centre
- Patients might be considered for CSII if:
  - uncontrolled glycaemia with conventional regimens
  - impaired awareness of hypoglycaemia
  - severe early morning hyperglycaemia ('dawn phenomenon')
  - pregnancy
  - extreme insulin sensitivity
  - particularly irregular or difficult lifestyle
  - aversion to multiple daily injections
- CSII can provide individualised programmed and self-adjustable infusions to coincide with the normal physiological pattern of insulin delivery more closely than injection regimens
- Several different types of infusion pumps with different capabilities and facilities are now available, including integrated glucose monitoring
- The procedures for use of CSII are outside the scope of this book

Education programmes

- Introduction of insulin must be accompanied by adequate educational support
- Explain general principles of insulin therapy: need, advantages, precautions, necessary and advised lifestyle adjustments
- Discuss available options for administration regimen
- Review range of injection devices
- Familiarise patient with the chosen device and insulins
- Demonstrate meticulously the injection technique with rotation of injection sites
- Consider in detail lifestyle implications, particularly meal composition and timing, use of snacks and adjustments with exercise
- Ensure awareness of hypoglycaemia, precautions and responses
- Empower patient to confidently manage SMBG and adjustments of insulin dose during changes in daily routine, common inter-current conditions and special situations such as driving and holidays
- Consider participation in a structured education programme eg. DAFNE or DESMOND, and expert patient group or other support activities

Patient self-mixing of insulins

To self-mix insulins:
- First draw up the rapid/short-acting preparation into the syringe
- Secondly draw up the intermediate/long-acting preparation
- Mix and inject

Note:
  - glargine and detemir can not be mixed with other insulins
  - lispro can not be self-mixed with other insulins but is available as pre-mixed Humalog

Storage of insulin

- Insulin is normally stored long-term at 4-8°C in a 'fridge
- Do not freeze-thaw insulin
- During use keep at room temperature or in a cool place, usually suitable for 1 month
- Avoid direct exposure to sun and temperatures above 25 °C

Taking insulin from a vial

- Shake vial gently and invert
- Draw air into syringe to injection volume required
- Pierce vial cap with needle
- Expel air into vial
- Draw insulin dose into syringe from inverted vial
- Check and expel any air bubbles by tapping syringe
- Slightly pinch skin at injection site to raise if preferred
- Insert needle at 45-90° to skin surface and inject syringe content

Pen injection device

- Check pen is loaded with cartridge and shake gently
- Dial 2 units and expel before use to remove air bubbles
- Dial required dose
- Slightly pinch skin at injection site if preferred
- Insert needle at 45-90° to skin surface and depress plunger

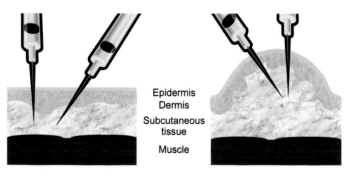

Figure 13.5 Injection technique

Timing of injections

- *Rapid-acting*
    - inject immediately before, during or soon after meal
- *Short-acting*
    - inject ~30 min (up to 60 min) before meal (delayed meal incurs risk of hypoglycaemia)
- *Intermediate-acting*
    - inject pre-breakfast and/or pre-evening meal
- *Long-acting*
    - inject pre-breakfast or pre-evening meal, or any defined time within a regular daily routine

Injection sites

- Subcutaneous injection sites are the abdomen, thigh, upper/outer buttocks and upper arm
- Rotation of sites avoids lipohypertrophy or lipoatrophy
- Advise to use similar injection sites at similar times each day for consistency of insulin profile
- Absorption rate is generally more rapid from abdomen than other subcutaneous sites
- Absorption rate is increased with exercise, raised temperature or other vasodilatatory situations or if injection site is massaged or injection is delivered into underlying muscle
- Areas of lipohypertrophy and lipoatrophy are prone to inconsistent insulin absorption
- Bruising can occasionally occur: try modifying injection technique
- Remind patient that different insulins are designed to have different rates of absorption

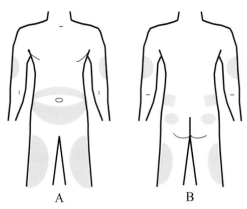

Figure 13.6 Subcutaneous insulin injection sites on front (A) and rear (B) of body

Table 13.8 Efficacy of insulin	
↓ HbA1c	variable
↓ FPG	variable
↓ PPG	variable
Other	The insulin dose and regimen can usually be adjusted to achieve (or nearly achieve) the desired target, but this may require subtle manipulation to avoid hypoglycaemia
	Hypoglycaemia can sometimes limit dose titration and prevent desired target being achieved or maintained
	Insulin dose requirement increases with the extent of insulin resistance, especially evident in *type 2 diabetes*

Contra-indications

- There are no absolute contra-indications for the use of some form of insulin replacement in *type 1 diabetes*
- Contra-indications may exist or develop for use of particular types of insulins and dosing strategies, but insulin therapy is mandatory for *type 1 diabetes*

- Insulin must be adopted if this is the last option for *type 2 diabetes*
- Adjustments of lifestyle to accommodate insulin therapy may be obligatory (however nicely they are broached)
- Type, dose, timing and regimen for insulin administration require careful consideration in patients with co-morbidities, especially significant kidney or liver disease, visual impairment, and conditions that impair mental faculties or require carer assistance
- Hypersensitivity or allergy are usually related to excipients or impurities, indicating a need to change insulin
- In very rare conditions with mutated and non-responsive insulin receptors, IGF-1 therapy is used

Adverse effects

- ***Hypoglycaemia***
    - more frequent in *type 1 diabetes*
    - more often severe in *type 1 diabetes*
    - more frequent with long-term duration of disease
    - more frequent with intensified basal-bolus regimen
    - persistent problem necessitates treatment revision
    - symptoms can occur at higher blood glucose concentrations than in non-diabetic individuals
        - this probably reflects conditioning to higher glucose levels in diabetes
        - counter-regulatory mechanisms become compromised in long-term diabetes

    Usual causes of hypoglycaemia are:
    - missed, delayed or smaller meal
    - unscheduled exercise
    - forgotten to carry or consume snack
    - changed daily routine
    - travel
    - excess alcohol
    - neglectful lifestyle
    - taken medication twice

Clinical causes of hypoglycaemia might be:
- need to change drug doses or regimen
- eating or malabsorption disorders
- recent change from animal to human insulin
- decreased metabolism of insulin-releasing drugs
- decreased renal or hepatic function
- other endocrine disorder affecting insulin sensitivity, eg. hypothyroidism, hypopituitism, Addison's disease

Hypoglycaemia unawareness
- can occur in long-term diabetes, possibly reflecting conditioning to frequent episodes of low blood glucose
- serious imposition and contra-indication for driving and other activities that impinge on personal or public safety

Noctural hypoglycaemia
- often unrecognised
- symptoms include morning headache and persistent tiredness after sleep
- often found in otherwise well controlled patients
- requires adjustment of dose, timing or type of evening medication
- can sometimes be controlled with changes in routine such as modification of bedtime snack or reduced alcohol

Weight gain
- typically 2-4 kg levelling after 6-12 months but can continue in type 2 patients
- may partly reflect decreased urinary glucose loss and anabolic effects of insulin
- may be partly ameliorated with use of metformin and reduced insulin dose

Lipohypertrophy
- localised, usually firm excess of subcutaneous adipose tissue associated with frequent use of injection site
- may reflect adipogenic effect of local excess insulin
- can interfere with insulin absorption
- consider using other sites if possible

- *Lipoatrophy*
  - localised loss of subcutaneous adipose tissue associated with frequent use of injection site
  - probably due to immune response to impurities in injection
  - relatively uncommon now
- *Allergy*
  - local or generalised allergic reactions to insulin are rare
- *Antibodies*
  - development of antibodies to insulin analogues can occur but these do not usually interfere significantly with efficacy and usually diminish during continued long-term use

Table 13.9 Approximate frequency of episodes of severe hypoglycaemia in type 1 and type 2 diabetes*

	% patients reporting ≥ 1 severe event/yr
Type 1 diabetes	
<5 yr duration	10-30% **
>15 yr duration	20-60% **
Type 2 diabetes	
Insulin treated	0.1-3%
Long-acting sulphonylurea	0.1-2%

* Severe hypoglycaemia involving third party assistance
** Upper range mostly with intensified regimens

Precautions

- Monitor glucose periodically during and after dose titration or dose adjustment to check glycaemic control
- Ensure ongoing support through education, advice and empowerment for self-management

○ Monitor visual, renal and hepatic function; be vigilant for emergence of other co-morbidities especially macrovascular diseases and neuropathic complications

○ Patient reminders: carry identification, carry glucose, ensure family, friends and work colleagues appreciate how to assist if required

○ Provide pre-conception counselling if planning pregnancy

○ Lipohypertrophy and lipoatrophy require changes of injection site and/or insulin preparation

Table 13.10 Early signs and symptoms of hypoglycaemia

Signs and symptoms	Action required
Hunger	Eat some sugary food
Sweating, tremor, palpitations	Take glucose
Dizzy, drowsy, uncoordinated, speech difficulty, impaired cognitive function, headache, nausea, malaise	Take glucose Seek assistance
Confusion, reduced consciousness, coma	Third party or medical intervention required

Drug interactions

○ Additional antidiabetic medications or other agents with intrinsic glucose-lowering activity will alter glycaemic control. These may predispose to hypoglycaemia and warrant adjustment to the insulin regimen or dose

- *type 1 diabetes*: such interactions focus on agents increasing insulin sensitivity or reducing counter-regulation
- *type 2 diabetes*: is also affected by agents that promote insulin release

○ Concurrent medication with intrinsic hyperglycaemic activity may require an increased insulin dose and occasionally necessitate an intensification of the regimen

Table 13.11 Potential drug interactions that could alter glycaemic control in insulin-treated patients	
Intrinsic glucose-lowering activity	Other antidiabetic drugs Salicylates (high dose)* Monoamine oxidase inhibitors* Some quinolone antibacterials* Alcohol
Intrinsic hyperglycaemic activity	Glucocorticoids, catecholamines, glucagon, growth hormone, high-dose thyroid hormones, some atypical antipsychotics, some diuretics
Beta adrenergic blockers can mask symptoms of hypoglycaemia and reduce counter-regulation	
* mainly in type 2 patients.	

Discontinue therapy

- Do not discontinue insulin completely
- If a meal is missed and the bolus injection has not been taken, then omit the bolus but continue basal insulin, take a snack if possible and continue daily routine at next meal
- If substantially reduced food intake reduce bolus insulin dose accordingly but continue basal insulin
- If unable to eat due to intercurrent illness omit bolus insulin, monitor glucose and reduce basal insulin if required. Note that some types of illness (eg. infections) can increase counter-regulatory hormones and increase basal insulin requirement
- If taken bolus (rapid/short-acting) insulin injection and then unable to eat meal, either take a snack or take emergency glucose, and inform someone responsible about dealing with a hypo

Driving

- In the UK and other European countries drivers with diabetes are required to declare their diabetes to the relevant regulatory authority. In the UK this is the Driver and Vehicle Licensing Agency (DVLA), Swansea.
- Advise patients that they must inform the DVLA if they:
    - are on insulin
    - have visual impairment
    - have problems with circulation or sensation in the legs
- The DVLA will take into account if the patient is receiving treatment that is prone to cause rapid onset or severe hypoglycaemia (eg. insulin, sulphonylurea), or if significant co-morbidity occurs (eg. visual impairment) or there is hypoglycaemia unawareness
- Before starting a journey, patients receiving medication that could precipitate hypoglycaemia are advised to:
    - check blood glucose and test regularly (every 2 h)
    - ensure that they are carrying adequate snacks
    - plan journey to allow adequate breaks

Insulin therapy precludes bus and train driving, and is only now considered for heavy goods vehicles in exceptional cases

Self-monitoring blood glucose (SMBG)

- SMBG is an important part of the patient education and empowerment process
- It is beyond the scope of this book to review the various devices
- SMBG should not be obsessive. It is important to assist drug dose titration or other drug adjustments, and it should be used by the patient to maintain a check on glycaemic control and facilitate full participation in a normal daily routine and to cope with changes to that routine.

Table 13.12 Characteristics of basal insulin preparations

Name	Manufacturer	Delivery	When administered*	Onset (h)	Peak (h)	Duration of action (h)
LONG ACTING						
Analogue						
Lantus (glargine)	Sanofi-Aventis	Vial, cartridge, pre-loaded pen	Anytime od sometimes bd	2-4	4-20	24+
Levemir (detemir)	Novo Nordisk	Vial, cartridge, pre-loaded pen	od/bd	2-4	6-8	18-24
Lente						
Hypurin bovine lente	Wockhardt	Vial	od, sometimes bd	2-6	8-12	18-24+
Hypurin Bovine Protamine Zinc	Wockhardt	Vial	od	4-8	8-20	24+
INTERMEDIATE ACTING						
Human						
Humulin I	Lilly	Vial, cartridge, pre-loaded pen	od/bd	1	2-8	10-16
Insulatard	Novo Nordisk	Vial, cartridge, pre-loaded pen	od/bd	1	2-12	16-22
Insuman Basal	Sanofi-Aventis	Vial, cartridge, pre-loaded pen	od/bd	1	2-4	12-18
Animal						
Hypurin Bovine Isophane	Wockhardt	Vial, cartridge	od/bd	1-4	6-12	16-22
Hypurin Porcine Isophane	Wockhardt	Vial, cartridge	od/bd	1-4	6-12	16-22

*30 min before a meal or at bedtime, once or twice a day

Table 13.13 Characteristics of bolus insulin preparations

Name	Manufacturer	Delivery	When administered	Onset	Peak (h)	Duration of action (h)
SHORT ACTING						
Human						
Actrapid	Novo Nordisk	Vial, cartridge, pre-loaded pen	15-30min before meal	30min	2-3	6-8
Humulin S	Lilly	Vial, cartridge, pre-loaded pen	15-30min before meal	30min	2-3	6-8
Insuman Rapid	Sanofi-Aventis	Vial, cartridge, pre-loaded pen	15-30min before meal	30min	2-3	6-8
Animal						
Hypurin Bovine Neutral	Wockhardt	Vial, cartridge	15-30min before meal	~1h	2-5	6-8
Hypurin Porcine Neutral	Wockhardt	Vial, cartridge	15-30min before meal	~1h	2-5	6-8
RAPID ACTING						
Analogue						
Apidra (glulisine)	Sanofi-Aventis	Vial, cartridge, pre-loaded pen	0-15min before or during meal	10min	1-2	3-4
Humalog (lispro)	Lilly	Vial, cartridge, pre-loaded pen	0-15min before or during meal	10min	1-2	3-4
NovoRapid (aspart)	Novo Nordisk	Vial, cartridge, pre-loaded pen	0-15min before or during meal	10min	1-3	3-4

Table 13.14 Characteristics of biphasic insulin preparations

Name	Manufacturer	Delivery	When administered	Onset	Peak (h)	Duration of action (h)
RAPID-INTERMEDIATE ACTING						
Analogue						
NovoMix 30 30 aspart:70 protamine	Novo Nordisk	Cartridge, pre-loaded pen	0-15min before or during meal	10min	1-4	10-20
Humalog Mix25 25 lispro:75protamine	Lilly	Cartridge, pre-loaded pen	0-15min before or during meal	10min	1-4	10-20
Humalog Mix50 50 lispro:50 protamine	Lilly	Pre-loaded pen	0-15min before or during meal	10min	1-4	10-20
SHORT-INTERMEDIATE						
Human						
Mixtard 30 30 soluble:70 protamine	Novo Nordisk	Vial, cartridge, pre-loaded pen	15-30min before meal	30min	1-8	10-20
Humulin M3 30 soluble:70 protamine	Lilly	Vial, pre-loaded pen	15-30min before meal	30min	1-8	10-20
Insuman comb 15 15 soluble:85 protamine	Sanofi-Aventis	Pre-loaded pen	15-30min before meal	30min	1-6	10-20
Insuman comb 25 25 soluble:75 protamine	Sanofi-Aventis	Vial, cartridge, pre-loaded pen	15-30min before meal	30min	1-6	10.20
Insuman comb 50 50 soluble:50 protamine	Sanofi-Aventis	Cartridge, pre-loaded pen	15-30min before meal	30min	1-6	10-20
Animal						
Hypurin porcine 30/70 mix 30 pork:70 protamine	Wockhardt	Vial, cartridge	15-30min before meal	30min	4-12	18-24

124

14 DIABETIC EMERGENCIES

Emergency procedures

This section provides summary protocols for the treatment of diabetic emergencies.

Diabetic ketoacidosis

Presentation
Dehydration, hypotension, tachycardia, hyperventilation, polyuria, polydipsia, ketotic breath, abdominal discomfort, recent weight loss, weakness, lethargy, drowsiness, coma in severe cases.

Check
Immediate: blood glucose, electrolytes, urea, osmolality, arterial pH and gases, urine ketones. Full blood count, amylase and blood/urine cultures.

Treatment of diabetic ketoacidosis
Start continuous iv administration of insulin, fluids and potassium.

Fluids
Depending on extent of dehydration, age and co-morbidities,

If plasma Na^+ < 155 mmol/L
  → infuse normal saline (150 mmol/L; 0.9%)
If plasma Na^+ > 155 mmol/L
  → infuse hypotonic saline (75 mmol/L; 0.45%)
  → after 2-3 h revert to normal saline
When blood glucose falls to <15 mmol/L (270 mg/dL)
  → add 5% glucose.
If pH < 7.0
  → consider adding sodium bicarbonate (600 mL of 1.26%)

Infusion rate
1 litre/h for first 2-3 h
Reduce thereafter to 1 litre/4-8h (3-6 litre over next 24 h)

Insulin

Continuous iv insulin infusion

Starting dose 5-10 Units/h   [children 0.1 Units/kg/h]
  → monitor glucose every 30 min

When glucose falls to <15 mmol/L (270 mg/dL)
  → reduce insulin dose to 1-4 Units/h
    [children ~0.02-0.05 Units/kg/h]

Monitor glucose every hour
  → reduce insulin dose as glucose normalises

Continue insulin dose 1-4 Units/h until stable normoglycaemia is achieved and patient is able to eat

Potassium

If plasma K⁺< 3.5 mmol/L .... add 40 mmol/L KCl
If plasma K⁺ = 3.5-5.5 mmol/L .... add 20 mmol/L KCl
If plasma K⁺ > 5.5 mmol/L .... no need to add KCl

Additional actions

* Treat any recognised precipitating causes or complications other than missed insulin eg. infection, MI, thromboembolism
* Ventilate with oxygen if respiratory distress
* Risk of cerebral oedema: consider iv mannitol or dexamethasone

Diabetic hyperosmolar non-ketotic state (HONK)

Presentation
Severe dehydration, hypotension, tachycardia, polyuria, polydipsia, weakness, impaired consciousness, coma in severe cases

Check
Immediate: blood glucose, electrolytes, urea, osmolality, arterial pH and gases, urine ketones. Full blood count and blood/urine cultures.

Treatment of HONK
Start continuous iv administration of insulin, fluids and potassium.

Fluids

Depending on extent of dehydration, age and co-morbidities,

If plasma Na^+ < 155 mmol/L

→ infuse normal saline (150 mmol/L; 0.9%)

If plasma Na^+ > 155 mmol/L

→ infuse hypotonic saline (75 mmol/L; 0.45%)

After 1h revert to normal saline

When blood glucose falls to <15 mmol/L (270 mg/dL)

→ add 5% glucose.

Infusion rate

1 litre/h for first 2-3 h

Reduce thereafter to 1 litre/4-8h (3-6 litre over next 24 h)

Insulin

Continuous iv insulin infusion

Starting dose 6 Units/h.

→ monitor glucose every 30 min

When glucose falls to <15 mmol/L (270 mg/dL)

→ reduce insulin dose to 1-4 Units/h

Monitor glucose every hour

→ reduce insulin dose as glucose approaches normoglycaemia

Continue insulin dose 1-4 Units/h until stable normoglycaemia is achieved and patient is able to eat

Potassium

If plasma K^+ < 3.5 mmol/L .... add 40 mmol/L KCl

If plasma K^+ = 3.5-5.5 mmol/L .... add 20 mmol/L KCl

If plasma K^+ > 5.5 mmol/L .... no need to add KCl

Additional actions

- Treat any recognised precipitating causes or complications other than missed insulin eg. infection, MI, thromboembolism
- Due to high risk of thromboembolic disease, anticoagulation with low molecular weight heparin is usually required
- Ventilate with oxygen if respiratory distress
- Risk of cerebral oedema: consider iv mannitol or dexamethasone.

Lactic acidosis

Presentation
Often non-specific, general malaise, hyperventilation, hypotension, vomiting, abdominal discomfort, hypothermia, myalgia, drowsy (known diabetes, features of metabolic acidosis but without ketonuria or significant dehydration)

Check
Immediate: blood glucose, lactate, electrolytes, arterial pH and gases. Full blood count and blood/urine cultures.

Diagnosis
Arterial lactate > 5 mmol/L
Arterial pH   < 7.25
Anion gap   > 15 mmol/L

Treatment of lactic acidosis
* Hospitalisation: intensive care
* Check medication, stop metformin
* If metformin excess suspected consider prompt haemodialysis
* Bicarbonate often used to correct the acidosis

Hypoglycaemia

Presentation
Sweating, tremor, headache, uncoordinated, nausea, malaise, drowsy, confused, impaired consciousness, coma and convulsions in severe cases

Check
Immediate: blood glucose

Treatment of hypoglycaemia
If sufficiently conscious:
 10-20 g glucose, eg ~3-6 dextrose tablets, or
 2-4 teaspoons of sugar, or 60-115 mL of Lucozade, repeat at intervals as required

If significantly impaired consciousness:

   buccal glucose gel, eg. Glucogel

If comatose:

   Either

      im injection 1 mg glucagon: give glucose if glucagon not effective in 10 min (do not use glucagon for sulphonylurea-induced hypoglycaemia)

   or

      iv injection 20% dextrose up to 50mL slowly

   or

      iv infusion 20% dextrose, typically 100mL

Subsequent glucose administration may be required if hypoglycaemia is caused by overdose of long-acting insulin or long-acting sulphonylurea

If recovery is delayed reconsider alternative cause of impaired consciousness, eg. stroke, other drug over-dose, excess alcohol

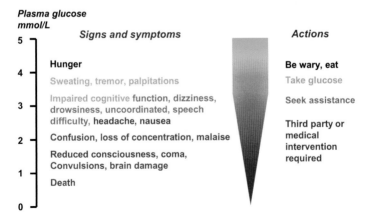

Figure 14.1 Typical signs and symptoms of hypoglycaemia in diabetic patients as plasma glucose falls.

15 REFERENCE MATERIAL

Glucose-lowering agents other than insulin

Class/ agent	Starting dose	Max dose	Duration of action[a] (h)	Metabolites	Elimination
Oral					
Biguanide					
Metformin	500-850 mg od	3000 mg	6-8	-	U ~100%
Metformin SR[b1]	500 mg od	2000mg	18-24	-	U ~100%
Sulphonylureas					
Chlorpropamide[c]	100 mg od	500 mg	>24	Active	U >90%
Glibenclamide	2.5 mg od	15 mg	18-24	Active	B >50%
Gliclazide	40 mg od	320 mg	12-20	Inactive	U ~65%
Gliclazide MR[b2]	30 mg od	120 mg	~24	Inactive	U ~65%
Glimepiride	1 mg od	6mg	18-24	Active	U ~60%
Glipizide	2.5 mg od/bd	15 mg	6-16	Inactive	U ~70%
Tolbutamide	500 mg od/bd	2000 mg	6-12	Inactive	U ~100%
Meglitinides					
Repaglinide	0.5 mg bd/tds,ac	16 mg	1-6	Inactive	B ~90%
Nateglinide	60 tds,ac	540 mg	1-4	Inactive	U ~80%
Gliptins (DPP-4 inhibitors)					
Sitagliptin	100 mg od	100mg	~24	Inactive[d]	U ~79%
Vildagliptin	50 mg bd	100 mg	~24	Inactive[e]	U ~85%
Thiazolidinediones					
Pioglitazone	15 mg od/bd	45 mg	~24	Active	B ~55%
Rosiglitazone	4 mg od/bd	8 mg	~24	Inactive	U ~65%
Alpha-glucosidase inhibitor					
Acarbose	50 mg bd/tds,ac	600 mg	~6	Inactive	I ~50%
Injectable/subcutaneous					
GLP-1 agonists					
Exenatide	5μg bd	20μg	4-6	Inactive	U
Liraglutide	0.6-1.2 mg od	1.8 mg	18- 24	Inactive	B/U

[a] Different formulations affect pharmacokinetics, timing of doses and duration of action.
[b1] Glucophage SR and [b2] Diamicron MR are modified release formulations that extend duration of action.
[c] Not used to initiate sulphonylurea therapy; being phased out.
[d] Mostly eliminated unchanged in the urine
[e] One slightly active metabolite.
[f] take with meals rich in complex carbohydrate
ac before meals; od once daily, bd twice daily; tds three times daily; ~ approximately;
B bile; I intestine; U urine.

Summary of action profiles of insulins

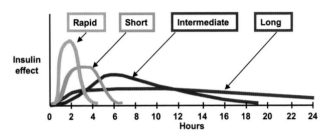

Approximate calculations

- **Plasma osmolality (mOsmol/L) =**
  2 x (plasma [Na$^+$] + plasma [K$^+$]) + plasma [glucose] + plasma [urea]
  - all plasma values measured in mmol/L
  - normal plasma osmolality 285-300 mOsmol/L

- **Plasma anion gap =**
  [Na$^+$] – [Cl$^-$ + HCO$_3^-$]
  - all plasma values measured in mmol/L
  - normal plasma anion gap < 15 mmol/L

- **Estimated glomerular filtration rate (eGFR)**
  Based on serum creatinine (μmol/L) using MDRD equation
  eGFR (mL/min/1.73m^2)

  = 186 x (creatinine in μmol/L)$^{-1.154}$ x (age in yrs)$^{-0.203}$

  [above x 0.742 for females]

- **Estimated creatinine clearance rate**
  Based on serum creatinine (μmol/L) using Cockcroft-Gault equation
  Creatinine clearance (mL/min)

  $$= \frac{(140 - \text{age in yrs}) \times \text{weight in kg} \times \text{gender constant}}{\text{Serum creatinine} (\mu\text{mol/L})}$$

  Gender constant: 1.23 for men; 1.04 for women

- **Friedewald equation***

$$LDLc = TC - (HDLc + \frac{TG}{2.2})$$ Values in mmol/L

* Inappropriate if TG > 4.5 mmol/L

- **Comparisons of units for lipids**

Lipid	Desirable values mmol/L	Conversion factor	Desirable values mg/dL
Cholesterol (TC)	< 4	x 38.6	< 155
LDL-c	< 2	x 38.6	< 80
HDL-c	> 1	x 38.6	> 40
Triglyceride	< 1	x 88.5	< 89

- **Child-Pugh score for chronic liver failure**

Points per feature	Total bilirubin μmol/L	Serum albumin g/L	INR	Ascites	Hepatic encephalopathy
1	< 34	> 35	< 1.7	Absent	None
2	34-50	28-35	1.71-2.2	Mild	Controlled by treatment
3	> 50	< 28	> 2.2	Severe	Uncontrolled by treatment

Class	Points (total)	1 yr survival
A	5-6	100%
B	7-9	81%
C	10-15	45%

- **Comparison of units for hormones**

Hormone	Reference range	Conversion factor	Alternative units
Insulin (fasting)	15-130 pmol/L	÷ 6.6	2-20 μUnit/mL
Glucagon (fasting)	< 50 pmol/L	x 3.4	< 170 pg/mL
Thyroxine T4	70-140 nmol/L	÷ 12.9	5-10 μg/dL
Triiodothyronine T3	1-3 nmol/L	÷ 0.015	65-200 ng/dL

- **Chronic kidney disease (CKD) stages**

Stage	eGFR mL/min/1.73m^2	Comment on kidney function
1	≥ 90	Normal
2	60-89	Mild reduction
3	30-59	Moderate reduction
4	15-29	Severe reduction
5	< 15	Very severe reduction or ESRD

- **New York Heart Association (NYHA)**

Classes of cardiac failure	
Class I	High risk but no apparent symptoms
Class II	Symptoms emerging during mild exertion, comfortable at rest
Class III	More marked symptoms during mild exertion, symptoms are limiting, comfortable at rest
Class IV	Severely symptomatic, discomfort with any exertion, symptoms occur at rest

- ## Comparisons of units for glucose and HbA1c measurements

Glucose	
mmol/L	mg/dL
17	306
16	288
15	270
14	252
13	234
12	216
11	198
10	180
9	162
8	144
7	126
6	108
5	90
4	72
3	54
2	36
1	18

HbA1c	
%	mmol/mol
12	108
11.5	103
11	97
10.5	92
10	86
9.5	81
9	75
8.5	70
8	64
7.5	59
7	53
6.5	48
6	42
5.5	37
5	31
4.5	26
4	20

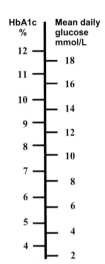

HbA1c % / Mean daily glucose mmol/L

- ## Calculator for BMI (kg/m²).

$$\text{Body mass index} = \frac{\text{weight} \ (\text{kg})}{\text{height} \ (\text{m}^2)}$$

Weight (kg)

Height (metres)	50	55	59	64	68	73	77	82	86	91	95	100	105	109	114	Height (feet and inches)
1.8	14	16	17	18	19	21	22	23	24	26	27	28	30	31	32	6'2"
1.8	15	16	17	18	20	21	22	24	25	26	28	29	30	32	33	6'1"
1.8	15	16	18	19	20	22	23	24	26	27	29	30	31	33	34	6'0"
1.8	15	17	18	20	21	22	24	25	26	28	30	31	32	33	35	5'11"
1.7	16	17	19	20	22	23	24	26	27	29	31	32	33	34	36	5'10"
1.7	16	18	19	21	22	24	25	27	28	30	32	33	34	35	37	5'9"
1.7	17	19	20	22	23	25	27	28	30	32	34	35	36	38	39	5'7"
1.6	18	19	21	23	24	26	27	29	31	33	35	36	37	39	40	5'6"
1.6	18	20	22	23	25	27	28	30	32	34	36	37	38	40	42	5'5"
1.6	19	21	22	24	26	27	29	31	33	35	37	38	39	41	43	5'4"
1.6	19	21	23	25	27	28	30	32	34	36	38	39	41	43	44	5'3"
1.5	20	22	24	26	27	29	31	33	35	37	39	40	42	44	46	5'2"
1.5	20	23	25	26	28	30	32	34	36	38	40	42	43	46	47	5'1"
1.5	21	23	25	27	29	31	33	35	37	39	41	43	45	47	49	5'0"
1.5	22	24	26	28	30	32	34	36	38	40	42	44	47	49	51	4'11"
1.4	23	25	27	29	31	33	36	38	40	42	44	46	48	50	52	4'10"
	110	120	130	140	150	160	170	180	190	200	210	220	230	240	250	

Weight (lbs)

135

References

General aspects

American Diabetes Association. Standards of medical care in diabetes – 2009. Diabetes Care 2009; 32: suppl 1 S13-S61.

The Expert Committee on the diagnosis and classification of diabetes mellitus. Report of the Expert Committee on the diagnosis and classification of diabetes mellitus. Diabetes Care 1997; 20: 1183-97.

JBS2: Joint British Societies' guidelines on prevention of cardiovascular disease in clinical practice. Heart 2005; 91: suppl V 1-55

National Institute for Health and Clinical Excellence. Type 2 diabetes: newer agents. Short clinical guideline 87. NICE, London, 2009. *www.nice.org.uk/CG87*

National Institute for Health and Clinical Excellence. Clinical guideline G. Management of type 2 diabetes. Management of blood glucose. NICE, London, 2005.

National Institute for Health and Clinical Excellence. Clinical guideline H. Management of type 2 diabetes. Management of blood pressure and blood lipids. NICE, London, 2005.

Department of Health. Quality and Outcomes Framework. Changes and New Indicators for 2009/10. London, 2009

International Diabetes Federation Clinical Guidelines Task Force. Global guideline for type 2 diabetes. International Diabetes Federation, Brussels, 2005. 80pp.

Day C. Metabolic syndrome – or What you will: definitions and epidemiology. Diabetes Vasc Dis Res 2007; 4: 32-38.

Anti-obesity agents

Sacks FM et al. Comparison of weight-loss diets with different compositions of fat, protein and carbohydrates. N Engl J Med 2009; 360: 859-73.

Choussein S et al. Effect of antiobesity medications in patients with type 2 diabetes mellitus. Diabetes Obesity Metabolism 2009 in press.

Day C, Bailey CJ. Sibutramine update. Br J Diabetes Vasc Dis 2002; 2: 392-7.

Henness S, Perry CM. Orlistat: a review of its use in the management of obesity. Drugs 2006; 66: 1625-56.

General reviews of antidiabetic agents

Krentz AJ, Bailey CJ. Oral antidiabetic agents: current role in type 2 diabetes mellitus. Drugs 2005;65:385-411.

Krentz AJ, Patel MB, Bailey CJ New drugs for type 2 diabetes: What is their place in therapy? Drugs 2008; 68: 2131-62.

Bailey CJ. Antidiabetic drugs other than insulin. Encyclopedia of Molecular Pharmacology, 2nd edn. Offermans S, Rosenthal W (eds), Springer, Berlin, 2009. pp116-125. Doi 10,1007/978-3-540-38918-7_109

Metformin

Bailey CJ, Turner RC. Metformin. N Engl J Med 1996;334:574-9.

Bailey CJ, Campbell IW, Chan JCN et al. Metformin: the gold standard. Wiley, Chichester, 2007. 288pp.

Bailey CJ. Metformin: effects on micro and macrovascular complications in type 2 diabetes. Cardiovasc Drugs Ther 2008; 22: 215-224.

Sulphonylureas and meglitinides

Groop LC. Sulfonylureas in NIDDM. Diabetes Care 1992; 15: 1737-54.

Rendell M. The role of sulfonylureas in the management of type 2 diabetes. Drugs 2004; 64: 1339-58.

Dornhorst A. Insulotropic meglitinide analogues. Lancet 2001; 358: 1709-15.

Blickle JF. Meglitinide analogues: a review of clinical data focused on recent trials. Diabetes Metab 2006: 32: 113-20

Thiazolidinediones

Yki-Jarvinen H. Thiazolidinediones. New Engl J Med 2004;351:1106-18.

Kahn SE, Haffner SM, Heise MA et al. Glycemic durability of rosiglitazone, metformin or glyburide monotherapy. N Engl J Med 2006; 355: 2427-43.

Nesto RW, Bell D, Bonow RO, et al. Thiazolidinedione use, fluid retention, and congestive heart failure: a consensus state-ment from the American Heart Association and the American Diabetes Association. Circulation 2003; 108: 294 1-8.

McGuire DK, Inzucchi SE. New drugs for the treatment of diabetes mellitus. Part 1. thiazolidinedione and their evolving cardiovascular impolications. Circulation 2008; 117; 440-9.

Dormandy JA, Charbonnel B, Eckland DJA et al. Secondary prevention of macrovascular events in patients with type 2 diabetes in the PROactive stydu (PROspective pioglitAzone Clinical Trial In macroVascular Events) : a randomised controlled trial. Lancet 2005; 366: 1279-89.

Incretins

Drucker DJ. The role of gut hormones in glucose homeostasis. J Clin Invest 2007; 117: 24-32.

Holst JJ. Glucagon-like peptide-1: from extract to agent. Diabetologia 2006;49 :253-60.

Flatt PR, Bailey CJ, Green BD. Recent advances in antidiabetic drug therapies targeting the enteroinsular axis. Curr Drug Metab 2009; 10: 125-137.

Amori RE, Lau J, Pittas AG. Efficacy and safety of incretin therapy in type 2 diabetes: systematic review and meta-analysis. JAMA 2007; 298: 194-206.

Campbell IW, Day C. Sitagliptin – enhancing incretin action. Br J Diabetes Vasc Dis 2007; 7: 134-9.

Croxtall JD, Keam SJ. Vildagliptin: a review of its use in the management of type 2 diabetes mellitus. Drugs 2008; 68: 2387-2409.

Acarbose

Lebovitz HE. Alpha-glucosidase inhibitors as agents in the treat-ment of diabetes. Diabetes Revs 1998; 6: 132-45.

Chiasson JL, Josse RG, Gomis R, et al. Acarbose for the prevention of diabetes mellitus: the STOP-NIDDM random-ised trial. STOP-NIDDM Trial Research Group. Lancet 2002;359; 2072-7.

Combinations

Bailey CJ.   Treating insulin resistance in type 2 diabetes with metformin and thiazolidinedione, Diabetes Obesity Metab 2005: 7: 675-91.

Bailey CJ, Day C. Fixed-dose single tablet antidiabetic combinations. Diabetes Obesity Metab 2009: 11: 527-33.

Insulin

Amiel SA, Dixon T, Mann R, Jameson K. Hypoglycaemia in type 2 daibetes. Diabetic Med 2008; 25: 245-54.

Bretzel RG, Nuber U, Landgraf W et al. Once-daily basal insulin glargine vs. thrice-daily prandial insulin lispro in people with type 2 diabetes on oral hypoglycaemic agents (APOLLO study). Lancet 2008; 371:1073-1084.

Douek IF, Allen SE, Ewings P et al. Continuing metformin when starting iNsulin in patients with type 2 diabetes: a double-blind randomized placebo-controlled trial. Diabetic Medicine 2005; 22: 634-40.

Garber AJ. Premixed insulin analogues for the treatment of diabetes mellitus. Drugs 2006; 66: 31-49.

Mooradian AD, Bernbaum M, Albert SG. Narrative review; a rational approach to starting insulin therapy. Ann Intern Med 2006; 145:125-34.

Hirsch IB. Insulin analogues. N Engl J Med 2005; 352: 174-83.

Holman RR, Thorne KI, Farmer AJ et al. Addition of Biphasic, Prandial, or Basal Insulin to Oral Therapy in Type 2 Diabetes. N Engl J Med 2008; 357:1716-30.

Plank J, Siebenhofer A, Berghold A et al. Systematic Review and Meta-analysis of Short-Acting Insulin Analogues in Patients With Diabetes Mellitus. Arch Intern Med 2005; 165: 1337-1344.

Raskin P, Allen E Hollander P et al. Initiating insulin therapy in type 2 diabetes: a comparison of biphasic and basal insulin analogs. Diabetes Care 2005; 28:260-265

Riddle MC, Rosenstock J Gerich et al. The treat-to-target trial: randomized addition of glargine or human NPH insulin to oral therapy of type 2 diabetic patients. Diabetes Care 2003; 26:3080-3086.

Sumeet R, Ahmad F, Lal A et al. Efficacy and safety of insulin analogues for the management of diabetes mellitus; a meta-analysis. Canadian Med Assoc J 2009; 180: 385-97.

White JR, Davis SN, Coopan R et al. Clarifying the role of insulin in type 2 diabetes management. Clinical Diabetes 2003; 21: 14-21.

16 IMAGES OF DIABETES THERAPIES

Metformin

Metformin
Glucophage

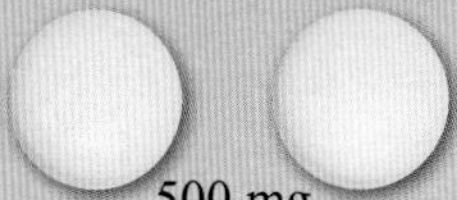

500 mg

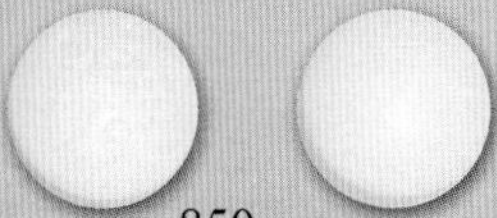

850 mg

Metformin
Glucophage SR

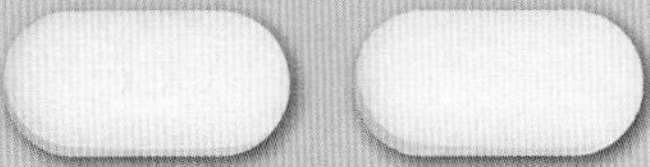

500 mg

Sulphonylureas

Glibenclamide
non-proprietary

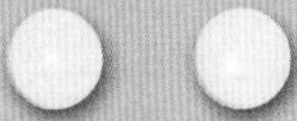

2.5 mg

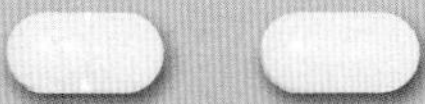

5 mg

Gliclazide
Diamicron

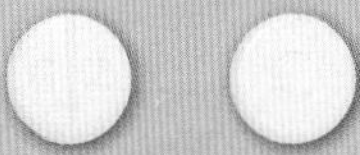

80 mg

Gliclazide
Diamicron MR

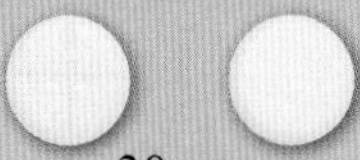

30 mg

Images shown are actual size

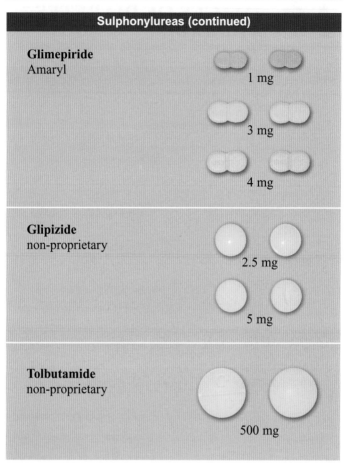

Sulphonylureas (continued)

Glimepiride
Amaryl

1 mg

3 mg

4 mg

Glipizide
non-proprietary

2.5 mg

5 mg

Tolbutamide
non-proprietary

500 mg

Images shown are actual size

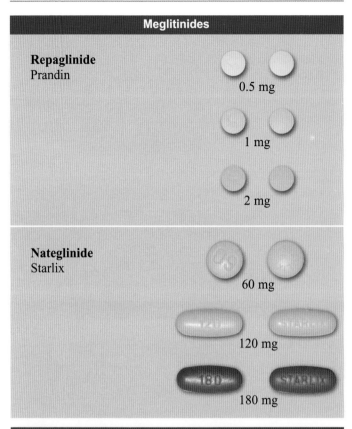

Meglitinides

Repaglinide
Prandin

0.5 mg

1 mg

2 mg

Nateglinide
Starlix

60 mg

120 mg

180 mg

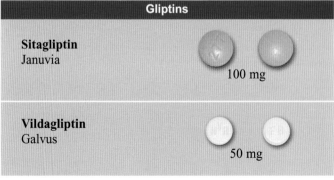

Gliptins

Sitagliptin
Januvia

100 mg

Vildagliptin
Galvus

50 mg

Images shown are actual size

Thiazolidinediones

Pioglitazone
Actos

15 mg

30 mg

Rosiglitazone
Avandia

4 mg

8 mg

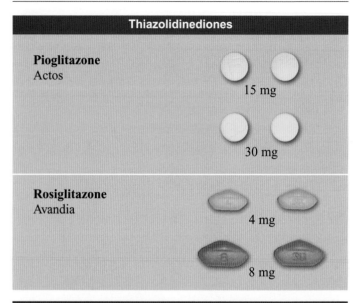

Acarbose

Acarbose
Glucobay

50 mg

100 mg

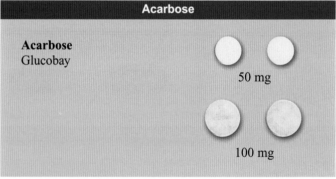

Images shown are actual size

Fixed-dose combinations

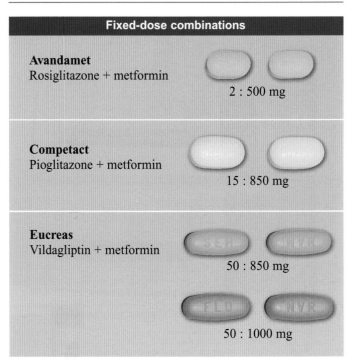

Avandamet
Rosiglitazone + metformin

2 : 500 mg

Competact
Pioglitazone + metformin

15 : 850 mg

Eucreas
Vildagliptin + metformin

50 : 850 mg

50 : 1000 mg

Images shown are actual size

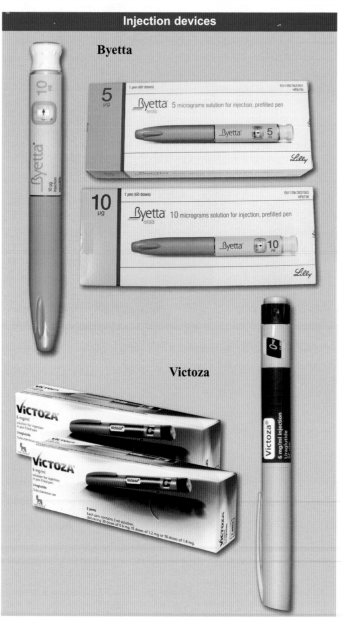

Images of GLP-1 agonist pens are shown half actual size

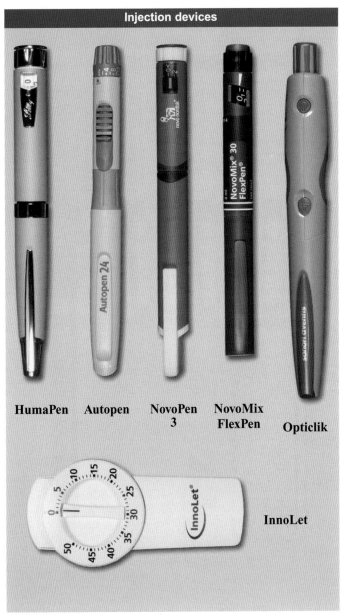

Injection devices

HumaPen   Autopen   NovoPen 3   NovoMix FlexPen   Opticlik

InnoLet

Diagrams shown are half actual size

Insulins and Insulin syringe

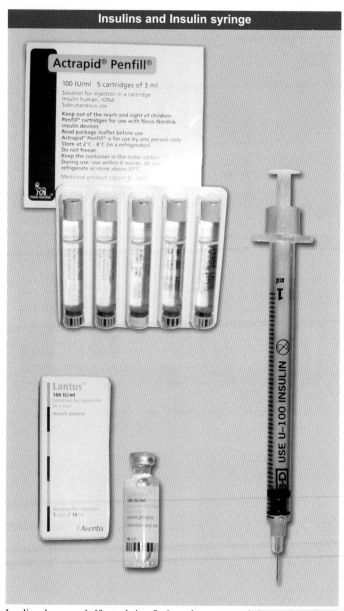

Insulins shown are half actual size, Syringe shown at actual size

INDEX

147

Index

Index